Master Cheng's
New Method
of Taichi Ch'uan
Self-Cultivation

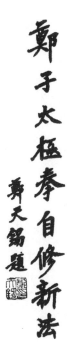

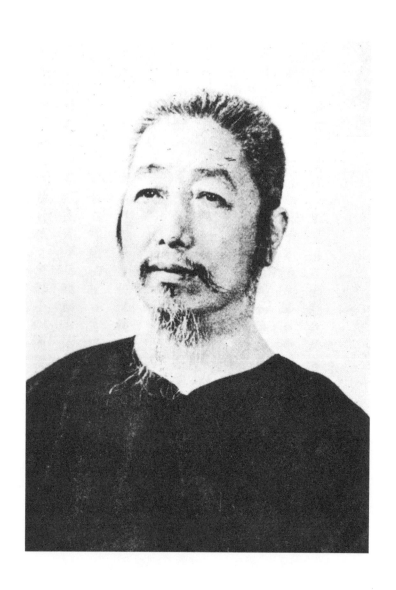

Master Cheng's New Method of Taichi Ch'uan Self-Cultivation

Cheng Man-Ch'ing

Translated by

Mark Hennessy

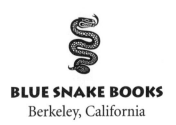

BLUE SNAKE BOOKS
Berkeley, California

Published by Blue Snake Books/Frog, Ltd.

Blue Snake Books/Frog, Ltd. books are distributed by
North Atlantic Books
P.O. Box 12327
Berkeley, CA 94712

Cover and book design by Paula Morrison
Printed in the United States of America
ISBN-13: 978-1-88331-992-2

North Atlantic Books' publications are available through most bookstores. For further information, call 800-337-2665 or visit our websites at www.northatlanticbooks.com and www.bluesnakebooks.com

Substantial discounts on bulk quantities are available to corporations, professional associations, and other organizations. For details and discount information, contact our special sales department.

Library of Congress Cataloging-in-Publication Data

Cheng, Man-ch'ing.
    [Cheng-tzu t'ai chi ch'üan tzu hsui hsin fa. English]
    Master Cheng's new method of T'ai Chi self-cultivation / by
Cheng Man-ch'ing : translated by Mark Hennessy.
        p.   cm.
    ISBN 1-883319-92-7 (alk. paper)
    1. T'ai chi ch'üan.   I. Hennessy, Mark.   II Title.
GV504.C51913   1999
613.7'148—dc21   99-11813
                                                               CIP

6   7   8   9   10   11   MALLOY   11   10   09   08   07   06

Table of Contents

Translator's Introduction

Professor Cheng Man-ch'ing composed his *New Method of Taichi Ch'uan Self-Cultivation* while in Taiwan during the early sixties in response to the many questions he received on the specifics of his "Simplified Thirty-Seven Posture Form" first presented in *Master Cheng's Thirteen Treatises on Taichi Ch'uan* of 1949. In that work, Cheng attempted to explain each posture as a defined response to a hypothetical attack. This complicated and hopelessly static format was employed previously by Cheng in the 1933 work he ghost-wrote for Yang Ch'eng-fu entitled *Uniting Form with Application in Taichi (T'i Yung Ch'uan Shu)*. As Cheng says below, he eventually came to understand the shortcomings of this presentation and in his *New Method* presents a detailed analysis of each move with only the practitioner in mind. His purpose herein is to describe the form with enough attention to detail so that a beginner with no previous experience could study and learn the postures solely through this book—hence the title "... *Self-Cultivation.*" Though this goal seems woefully impractical and wildly optimistic, the *New Method* is our most detailed account of the intricacies of Cheng's shortened form and it remains an important companion volume to any student's taichi study.

The origin of the Simplified Thirty-Seven Posture Form and its evolution, from its creation in 1938 to its publication in the late forties, is well known and described in almost every book published by or for Cheng. What is never addressed, however, is why Cheng chose the number thirty-seven. On page forty-nine of Chen Wei-ming's 1929 *Questions and Answers on Taichi Ch'uan*, this elder classmate of Cheng creates a shortened form based upon an earlier Thirty-Seven Posture Form of Hsu Hsuan-ping. In the mid-eighties, Cheng's last disciple and self-proclaimed heresiarch, Wu Kuo-chung, was busy divulging Cheng's esoteric teachings to all who cared to listen. One of these secrets was the reason why Cheng chose the number thirty-seven. He divulged that thirty-six postures (six squared) were chosen from the Long Yang Form and assigned an *I Ching* hexagram. The final "secret" thirty-seventh posture and hexagram (the enigma wrapped within a labyrinth!) was a Left-Hand Push hidden within the Shoulder Strike Posture.

Knowing Cheng's love of *I Ching* lore, but not his penchant for secrets, I asked Liu Hsi-heng for any clues to the origin of the number series. He replied that Cheng merely chose the postures, counted the numbers, and arrived at thirty-seven. He criticized Wu, saying, "After someone is dead anyone can propose numerous reasons for any single act. Moreover, the *I Ching* is large enough to support almost any belief."

I was yet intrigued by Wu's contention that Cheng did not create his Thirty-Seven Posture Form irrespective of the numerology involved. I placed Cheng's two Chinese taichi books together (the *New Method* and the *Thirteen Treatises*) and compared the postures with their assigned numbers. From the chart on the next page, it is clear that neither Liu nor Wu is correct. For though every posture has a different corresponding number and repetitious postures are counted differently, both sets arrive at thirty-seven.

If Wu was correct, each posture would be assigned a definitive number correlating to an *I Ching* hexagram and the Left-Hand Push within the Shoulder Strike would be counted as a

TABLE 1

Posture	Thirteen Treatises	New Method
Preparation	1	1
Beginning	2	*
Left Ward-Off	3	2
Right Ward-Off	4	3
Roll-Back	5	4
Press	6	5
Push	7	6
Single Whip	8	7
Lift Hands	9	8
Shoulder Strike	10	9
White Crane	11	10
Brush Left Knee, Twist Step	12	11
Strumming the Guitar	13	12
Step Forward, Block, Parry, Punch	14	13
Sealing, Closing	15	*
Cross Hands	16	14
Embrace Tiger	17	15
Rely on Fist below Elbow	18	16
Right Retreating Monkey	20	18
Left Retreating Monkey	21	19
Diagonal Flying	22	20
Cloud Hands Right	23	21
Cloud Hands Left	24	22
Squatting Single Whip	25	23
Right Golden Chicken	26	24
Left Golden Chicken	27	25
Separate Right Leg	28	26
Separate Left Leg	29	27
Turn the Body, Kick	30	28
Plant Fist	31	29
Fair Lady, one	32	30
Fair Lady, two	33	31
Fair Lady, three	*	32
Fair Lady, four	*	33
Seven Stars	34	34
Ride Tiger	35	35
Sweep Lotus	36	36
Shoot Tiger	37	37

separate number with its own hexagram. But it is evident that in the *New Method* Cheng grouped the Preparation Posture and the Beginning Posture together as a single number; while in the *Thirteen Treatises* he considers Step Forward, Block, Parry, and Punch as two separate postures. He then catches up with his numberings by curiously assigning Fair Lady four separate posture numbers. It is curious because all other repetitive postures are only assigned two numbers and referred to as simply the Right and Left versions—as in Cloud Hands and Repulse Monkey—though each is performed three to five separate times. If Liu was correct and Cheng was oblivious to the final number, the two sets should have yielded different results. In addition, it is commonly known that several nameless, numberless postures within the Simplified Form and employed by Cheng as transitional postures actually originated from the Long Yang Form, such as the move proceeding Right Golden Chicken and preceding Separate Right Leg.

To add to the confusion, on page 135 of Cheng's *Simplified Method of Calisthenics for Health and Self Defense* (Berkeley: North Atlantic Books, 1981), a third set of numberings for the solo form combines to forty-two postures—despite the fact that the form explanation in the work adheres to the *Thirteen Treatises* thirty-seven posture numberings.

In every book Cheng himself published, he manages to count the postures differently and yet makes absolutely sure that the final count is thirty-seven. None of this confusion bodes well for Wu Kuo-chung's claim of correlative cosmology. Thankfully, Wu's secrets, and his reputation, have since been relegated to the dustbin of useless, self-serving, contrived esoterica—and Wu himself remains adrift in a cup of water.

The question remains as to why Cheng labored in fitting his Simplified Form into an uncompromising thirty-seven-posture model. He never wrote of any reason, nor alluded to the possibility of a correlative cosmological interpretation. Without resorting to tactics like Wu Kuo-chung's shamanistic prognostications, the issue may never be resolved. Cheng did say, emulating Confucius, "I have no secrets." We can only assume that if this question was important he would have left us a clue. For though he never pandered to the student nor belabored a point, neither could he, a prodigious writer of classical Chinese and the author of three taichi books, be accused of hiding a jewel at the expense of the nation.

The language Cheng employs in his *New Method* is unique and requires some explanation. First, he creates the compound noun, waist/hip joint (*yau-k'ua*) for what is commonly, though erroneously, translated as waist. The hip joints assume a greater level of importance in later Cheng thought. My teacher once quoted the Professor as saying, "Whoever has the most relaxed hip joints has the best taichi!" Cheng's pursuit of relaxed hip joints found fruition in the exercise he entitled the "Constant Bear," translated in my *Cheng Man-Ch'ing: Master of Five Excellences*, (Berkeley: Frog Ltd., 1995). The Taichi Classics' admonition that the waist "appear boneless, as if it can fold over one hundred times" is directly related to this exercise. Moreover, none of Cheng's English books on taichi, including Robert Smith's, contain this noun compound.

Another word encountered herein, yet entirely absent from all of Cheng's English texts, is the verb form of the word "momentum." With reckless abandon for the English language, I have created the verb *momentate*, as this approximates the use employed by Cheng. In his form explanations, for example, he will write, "The arm momentates to the left rear...," meaning simply that the arm moves to the left rear through the momentum of the previous move. This conserves the energy needed to continually instigate impetus. Every movement, according to Cheng, produces momentum. And the true secret to a smooth-flowing taichi form is to redirect momentum back to movement—which then produces more movement and momentum.

It is interesting to note that Cheng is never explicit concerning weight distribution. The foot diagrams are our only source on whether the weight is in the 70/30 position or full/empty. Regardless of the weight distribution to the two legs, and even when the weight is shown to be shifted only to 70 percent full, he will always say, "Shift fully on to the leg, bend the knee, and sit on the leg." This seems to say that there are no static 70/30 weight distributions; everything is moving either to substantial or insubstantial—a position held by many close associates of Cheng, though he never admits this in writing. The foot diagrams were not drawn by Cheng; they are often confusing, and sometimes wrong.

The reader will note my original translation of traditionally mistranslated posture names. "Look at Fist under Elbow" is corrected as "Rely on Fist...." This prevents the practitioner from looking down at his fist. The Chinese character for "look" can also mean, as in English, "rely upon" as in the phrase, "We look to him ..." The posture commonly mistranslated as "Step Back to Repulse the Monkey" presents a ludicrous picture of someone stepping back to push away a monkey. The correct interpretation is not that you are stepping back, repulsing a monkey, but that you are a retreating, repulsing monkey. This posture originated in the Taoist Five Animal Frolics. Mr. Liu would often tell us to imagine ourselves performing this move like a circus monkey walking backwards, balanced atop a circus ball. The mistranslated "Step Forward to the Seven Stars" ignores the traditional teaching passed on by the Yang family of collectively referring to seven parts of the body (the head, shoulder, forearm, hip joint, knee, hand, and foot) as the "Seven Stars." Chang San'feng was called old "Seven Needle" most likely in reference to the dangerously sharp, martial qualities of his seven body points. This posture is therefore translated as "Seven Stars Step Forward." I fully realize I may be stepping forward onto some of my readers own sensitive toes by altering the cozy, misleading, mistranslated postures. I only hope they will notice how many traditionally, correctly translated postures I have kept, and allow me these few indulgences.

In order to save publishing costs, Cheng tacked his *Thirteen Treatises* on to the end of the *New Method*. He was then faced with the decision of either leaving the calligraphic frontpieces contributed by highly influential politicians stuck somewhere in the middle of two books, or switching the frontpieces written expressly for the *Thirteen Treatises* on to the *New Method*. Delicately balancing political allegiances, Cheng completely discards Wang's calligraphy (having been voted out of the legislature by that time); he switches Chiang Kai Shek's and Yu Yo Ren's calligraphy to the front of the New Method (having been Madame Chiang's painting teacher and a close confidant of Yu); and he leaves Chen Wei-ming's preface to stand alone in its original spot (Chen having died some twenty years earlier). I leave it to competent and comprehensive future translators of the *Thirteen Treatises* to translate these frontpieces and supply the political significance of their removal and displacement. My energies focused on the *New Method* alone.

Cheng entitles his work "... Self-Cultivation" but does he mean self-study? Or self-practice? Or self-teaching? I believe not. Cheng once remarked, "Practicing is easy, but true self-cultivation is rare," and throughout the work the reader gets the feeling that Cheng is more interested in cultivating the *sui generis* rather than the autodidact. My teacher and the editor of this work, Liu Hsi-heng, always kept the *New Method* close at hand and referred to it whenever questioned on the form. This book is the main reason he never authored any taichi form analysis or allowed any pictures or videos of himself to be taken. He always told us, "Professor Cheng's book and pictures are complete in themselves and are all you will ever need."

Taichi in the States is shedding its alternative connotations as it enters mainstream acceptance and the ranks of taichi prac-

titioners is steadily growing. But as we have grown up, we have
grown apart, separating into competing camps led by individual characters. Mistaken allegiances to masters and methods
have driven a wedge between people and through the heart of
the art. Just as no leaf turns yellow but with the silent knowledge of the entire tree, we must acknowledge our undeniable
interconnectedness with all taichi practitioners. How complete
will our art be if we practice to unify our body and ch'i while
our spirit is enmeshed in political alliances? One factor for dis-
association, however, remains constant and true. When men
cease to be relevant they study to be dowagers—usurpers of
title, conservators of writ. We must stand firm against the
monopoly of truth and the aristocracy of knowledge. The Tao
of taichi is not partisan nor its writings subject to an impri-
matur. Those who seek to monopolize taichi's illuminating
mirror view intrusions to their exclusive legitimacy through the
backside of a shattered mirror—of course they see nothing.
Turning it around, they see only their splintered reflection—
and then profess their diversity! Many practice taichi but true
inner self-cultivation is rare, and impossible, until we relax our
grip on that mirror of illumination and return to embrace and
assist one another.

Mark Hennessy
Chicago, 1997

Master Cheng's
New Method
of Taichi Ch'uan
Self-Cultivation

Ku Wei-Chun's Preface

CHENG MAN-CH'ING is one of China's most ardent scholars. Endowed with an astute intellect, his scholarly endeavors reveal a level of refinement and profundity in subjects as diverse as literature, calligraphy, painting, and medicine. Especially enlightening, however, is his exposition of taichi's theoretical principles of form and function. Though I have never, regretfully, asked him for directions in this field, I knew of his reputation for quite some time. I am also aware that his earlier work, *Thirteen Treatises on Taichi Ch'uan*, has gained welcome acceptance amongst my countrymen.

During the War of Resistance, Cheng was invited by the British Counsel General to give a demonstration of his martial art at a reception held in Chungking at the British Embassy. Attending the demonstration was a British military delegation, and two or three of the men accepted invitations to test themselves against Cheng. With but a raise of his arm and a turn of his body, Cheng sent every opponent tumbling several feet away. Cheng later held a demonstration at a reception for American forces stationed in Chungking, with much the same results. He then planned to have his *Thirteen Treatises on Taichi Ch'uan* translated into English to spread and broaden the art in Europe and America.

Currently, Mr. Cheng is temporarily residing in New York.

In addition to establishing classes and teaching lessons, he also travels to various venues to lecture and demonstrate taichi. All of this proves his passionate desire to introduce Chinese culture and art to the West.

Now he has authored *Master Cheng's New Method of Taichi Ch'uan Self-Cultivation,* where he collects, edits, and places before the public his cumulative experience culled from a lifetime of practice, together with theoretical principles developed from his profound studies. We sense in him a compassion and a fervent wish to share his goodness with all.

Therefore I have penned these few lines as a Preface.

1966
Ku Wei-chun of Wu Ling

Author's Introduction

PEOPLE CAN TALK about the Way to healthy living without ever understanding the truth of the matter. Perhaps Chuang Tzu's collected writings, with their emphasis on nourishing life, could be the Classic on Healthy Living. Upon examination, unfortunately, his recommendations for a healthy lifestyle are repetitions of mainstream Confucian values of conscientiousness in appetite and sexuality.[1] Neither school left any specific outline for realizing their beliefs.

Po Chi, the Supreme Teacher and protagonist in the *Yellow Emperor's Classic on Internal Medicine (Nei Ching)*, described men who followed the Way saying:

They escape the infirmities of age and remain healthy because essence and spirit are guarded within. At their zenith, their sinews harmonize with their vessels, marrow hardens their bones, and ch'i improves their circulation.

The Yellow Emperor compiled these and other teachings into his *Nei Ching*—the only true Classic for Healthy Living. The Taichi Classics, however, do express similar ideas, such as, "When ch'i is gathered within the bones, they become unbreakable," and, "Proceeding from understanding energy, rise to divine clarity." In fact, taichi manifests the principles of wisdom found not only in the *Nei Ching* and *I Ching*, but also Taoism and

5

Confucianism. It embraces every aspect of these philosophies, from the coarse to the refined and the superficial to the profound, while providing a practical application for the form. It is only due to the penetrating intelligence of taichi's creator, Chang San-feng, that the art rose to such profound levels.

There are some ignorant individuals in the world who foolishly believe they can skim off the cream of taichi and apply it to other martial arts, but they merely lack the capacity for serious study. It takes total dedication and a commitment to taichi alone to ever approach the level where your sinews harmonize with your vessels or marrow hardens your bones. Such profundities cannot be penetrated by a casual approach to taichi. I took up study of this art when my weakened body was about to breathe its last breath, and through it I was given a second chance in life. I have been practicing continuously for over forty years and have come to understand the principles expounded in the Taichi Classics; every word is concise, true, and encompassing.

Regardless of all these benefits, the Tao of taichi is still neglected. Some dismiss its self-defense applications as impractical; others seek only its physical or mental benefits. Each of taichi's postures has a particular application, just as every object casts a distinct shadow. Taichi form practice that ignores functional application bestows health benefits that are artificial at best.

Some proverbs advise teachers to withhold vital techniques or to teach only sons and not daughters. I do not trust such advice. Such selfish interests not only deprecates our national arts and culture, it paves the way for their complete disintegration. Remember the Yellow Emperor's advice on teaching:

> *Teaching an unworthy student may squander a divine gem, but dismissing a deserving pupil erodes the Tao.*[3]

I encourage all who follow this Way to exercise caution and discipline.

Eliminating Three Faults

M Y *New Method of Taichi Ch'uan Self-Cultivation* can help those pressed by work schedules, women busy with household chores, or any enthusiast whose remote location precludes him the opportunity for class study. It allows them to study my teachings in lieu of private correspondence. Though taichi encompasses both form and function, my *New Method* analysis details the finer points of the postures and defers any explanation about taichi's self-defense application. Readers interested in self-defense may refer to the last chapters of my *Simplified Method of Calisthenics for Health and Self Defense*, or to my *Thirteen Treatises*.

There are three basic faults you must eliminate before you begin to practice taichi on your own. My experience from over forty years of teaching has shown me that all successful students have eliminated these three faults, but only after constant practice and faithful devotion. If it is your fate to be a little dull, just work ten times harder than anyone else. The method to rid yourself of these faults is simple and accessible, but most people cling tenaciously to their bad habits and fail to take decisive, corrective action. As a young man I too had these faults and so can discuss them with some degree of familiarity.

The first fault is the lack of perseverance. Confucius once said that even the unorthodox arts of a sorceress required perseverance.[4] How much more important is it in taichi, which encompasses the principles of philosophy and science! Taichi's philosophy of the soft overcoming the hard and concentrating your ch'i for softness is based on the *I Ching*, the *Nei Ching*, and the *Tao Teh Ching*. Even the idea of moving a thousand pounds with four ounces of strength is simply an extension of the fulcrum principle as explained in science and the returning force of resistance as illustrated in dynamics. Taichi is the crystallization of philosophy and science and can bridge the gap separating the East from the West—bringing intercultural exchanges that benefit far more than merely the form and application of taichi alone. Studying taichi without perseverance will have you not only constantly grappling over the same problems, you will eventually exit this treasure trove empty-handed.

I always regret my lack of perseverance when young. I began to practice martial arts to strengthen my frail body but would invariably stop as soon as I felt the slightest bit better. Finally, thirty-nine years ago, bedridden with tuberculosis, I resolved to begin practicing and never stop again. At the time, I practiced the long taichi form and discovered that by hurrying I could whittle away six or seven minutes from the overall performance. I practiced every morning and night to ensure continuity and perseverance—though I was busy with teaching commitments and extracurricular activities. Every morning I practiced the form before I washed or ate; at night I went through one round before I slept. I made good progress and this routine soon developed into a daily habit. My philosophy of life was to joyfully assist others regardless of the personal sacrifice involved. How could I expect to benefit humanity if I lacked the perseverance to practice a few minutes every day to remain healthy? I despised my ignorance and was painfully determined to correct my error.

The second fault is greed. Do not bite off more than you can chew. Lao Tzu certainly understood this when he said, "Small amounts are understandable, too much is confusing."[5] When I was young, my friend Lu Chien once came to visit me. As he prepared to leave he said, "Ancient noblemen parted with gifts of words, and so I leave you with some parting advice. By continuing the tradition of your ancestral namesake, 'Cheng Ch'ien, Master of Three Excellences,' your talents may one day be equally acknowledged—but your obsession for learning may limit any future success. Heed my words! Concentrate on your efforts on poetry, calligraphy, and painting."[6] Today I owe every accomplishment to this beneficial friend and his kind advice. The *I Ching* said that what is easy will be easily understood; what is simple will be easily followed—and it is the same in taichi.[7] Quietly practice and memorize a few postures each session to avoid confusion.

In the spring of 1938, I was Director of the Hunan Martial Arts Academy. Everybody, both young and old, male and female, did some form of martial art—it seemed almost a requirement. To further promote taichi, I decided to personally teach the martial arts instructors from every county in a two-month taichi course. Since the long form could not be taught adequately in that time frame, I created the Simplified Form. Remember that taichi originally had only thirteen postures. Additional postures added on throughout the centuries made it too time-consuming to be popularly accepted. The age we live in dictates our necessities. So I merely reduced the number of postures to thirty-seven—still twenty-four more than the original! There are some misguided people who condemn my Simplified Form without understanding the hardships I have endured to promote this unparalleled art.[8] All I could do was continue quietly on. Though my form is called "simplified," it is not at all easy to learn.

I traveled to Shanghai after the war to visit my elder classmate, Ch'en Wei-ming, and show him the manuscripts of my *Thirteen Treatises*. He praised the work and wholeheartedly agreed with my ideas—he even offered to write an introduction.

Mr. Ch'en is a true scholar and would never support inferior work out of partiality to its author.

The third fault is impatience. Confucius once said that rushing forward obscures the goal—true words of wisdom![9] Emulate the stream that gradually forms its own watercourse rather than brutishly forging ahead. The ancients approached the literary arts in this manner.

> *Immersed and steeped in the lush richness of words.*
> *Savor their beauty, relish their glory.*

And:

> *Scattered through the breaking frost.*
> *Contented with my flowing thoughts.*[10]

I will venture to say that the same holds true for taichi. This art does not merely combine form with application or focus on mind/hand coordination. We must comprehend its philosophical basis and understand the practical application of its scientific principles—only then will its benefits be limitless. By following my ideas for eliminating these three faults, you can progress smoothly, quickly, and unimpeded.

Three Types of Fearlessness

THERE ARE ONLY a few reasons why anyone finds the impetus to study taichi as an exercise. Some are sick and study to regain their health, some are worried of being attacked and study to learn about self-defense, and some are intrigued by taichi's mystical subtleties and study to investigate their validity. Aside from these, many are merely following the trends of fashion, riding the current of the crowd, and lack perseverance. My discussion on fearlessness is intended only for those willing to exert effort.

First: Do not fear bitter work. If you do you will never progress. The Taichi Classics say that the proper root is in the foot.[11] A beginner can develop a root by simply spending three to five minutes, morning and night, standing fully on a single leg. Alternate legs and gradually increase the time while you sink lower. This bitter work not only develops a root, it stimulates the cardiovascular system, which benefits the brain. It is essential that your ch'i sinks to the tan-t'ien, both feet adhere to the floor, and you exert absolutely no force. When practicing this Standing Posture, you may assist your balance by lightly touching a chair or table with the middle and index fingers. After a while use only the index finger. When you can stand unassisted, you may choose either the Lift Hands Posture or Playing the Guitar Posture to continue your practice. The Single Whip

Posture develops openness and extension while the Preparation Posture cultivates undifferentiated unity.[12] These postures are essential in understanding taichi's form and application—so do not neglect them!

Second: Do not fear losing. The fundamental principle in taichi is: "Yield to follow others." Yielding up your position to follow your opponent is, most decidedly, losing. In Chapter One of my *Thirteen Treatises* I discussed the importance of investing in losing—but where do you begin? While listening to your opponent's advance and attack, not only should you not resist, you should not even consider a counterattack. Simply adhere and stick to him, then you can lightly turn and neutralize. The sensitivity required for this eludes those with a crude or superficial understanding. Moreover, a beginner cannot possibly avoid losing and defeat, so if you fear defeat you may as well not even begin. If you want to study, begin by investing in loss. An investment in loss eliminates any greed for superficial advantages. Greediness for petty advantages results in minor losses, while greediness for large advantages results in major losses. On the other hand, a tiny investment in loss brings minor benefits, while a large investment in loss brings you great long-term benefits.

The intelligent and sensitive realize a unification of form with function. Where do we start? With Lao Tzu's idea, taichi's prime directive is: "Concentrate your ch'i to become soft and young." Concentrating your ch'i to become soft is the only proper method to invest in loss—then you will not fear losing. The Taichi Classics says, "Let him attack with all he has, I will deflect it with four ounces of strength." At this level you have learned the application of softness.

Third: Do not fear ferocity. Lao Tzu described men who have cultivated the life principle saying: "A rhino finds no place to gore, a tiger feels nothing to claw, a soldier has nowhere to stab."[13] Why is this? Because they have no fear of death. So rather than praising the ferocity of a rhino, tiger, or weapon, Lao Tzu exalts the softness which overcomes all hardness. When you penetrate the basic principles of taichi you possess a spirit of great fearlessness. Nothing can harm you once you discard your sense of self, not soldiers nor rhinos. Fear tenses your body and spirit, and prevents you from relaxing—how then can you be soft? If you are not soft then you are hard. Mencius said to nourish your vast, flowing ch'i; Hsun Shih said to remain calm even before an avalanche.[14] Together their sentiments combine to emulate Lao Tzu's idea of concentrating your ch'i to become soft. Then no ferocity is frightful.

Speaking on My Experience

SEVERAL YEARS AGO, my student asked me, "You, sir, adroitly unite five distinct arts. From your lifetime of teaching, which art do you enjoy the most?" I replied, "Taichi brings me the most pleasure." One man was skeptical and asked, "Is not taichi a somewhat crude and simple art?" I replied, "Obviously you do not understand. Taichi is the crystallization of mankind's most profound philosophical ideals. Its subtle and essential elements raise it above every martial art, and makes perfection more elusive than any beaux-art." When asked to continue, I related the following.

When I was a young man of twenty, I taught classes in poetry, calligraphy, and painting. Calligraphy provided me the most pleasure because I had benefited from its strengthening and rejuvenative properties. As I approached my vigorous years, I drifted to Szechuan and kept food on my table by practicing herbal medicine. Quite to my surprise, I became a moderately famous herbalist—with some people even calling me a "savior of the world's living." My busy schedule left precious little time for food and rest; it pains me even now to remember those times. Greeted each morning by sorrowful, long faces—for my healthy patients never bothered to visit—I was shouldered with the responsibility of saving lives. When I teach taichi today, however, I still cure illnesses, prolong life, and gladden the spirit, but I can also enjoy the gathering of young and old, and the sharing of goodness with others.

> *Resembling Old Lai's childish antics,*
> *never retiring though aged.*
> *Surpassing Hua Tuo's animal frolics,*
> *always concentrating ch'i for softness.*

Herein, truly, lie health and happiness.

I have distilled my forty years of teaching experience into twelve simple words: Swallow the heavens ch'i; tap the earth's strength; prolong life through softness. Each of these three principles has a specific body point to develop ch'i.[15] Remember that ch'i is transported by blood, so that circulating your blood invigorates your ch'i.

First, the *ni-wan* point on top of your head can receive heaven's ch'i and thus stimulate your sensitive ch'i. Whenever you have time, hold your *ni-wan* erect, swallow, and sink heaven's ch'i to your tan-t'ien. Remember that heaven possesses an infinite amount of ch'i, so never feel greedy. This energy has tremendous health benefits.

Second, the *yung-ch'uan* point in the middle of your foot can tap into the earth's ch'i and provide you with rooting strength. Whether you are walking, sitting, or just standing, be aware that your feet adhere to the ground. Continue until you feel your feet almost sink into the ground and connect to the earth's gravitational pull. This too will develop a root. Remember that the earth supports vast amounts of strength. Tapping into but a fraction of what the earth can support will engender you with unlimited potential.

Third, the tan-t'ien point, midway between the other two points and near your waist, is where you concentrate your ch'i for softness. Remember that Lao Tzu believed that softness keeps us young. It makes the waist lively and flexible, which enriches our urogenital ch'i, which bestows longevity. So whether you are walking, standing, sitting, or sleeping, keep your mind and ch'i mutually on guard in the tan-tien—much as a mother hen guards over her eggs. This is the meaning of the phrases:

Know where to rest ... rest at the attainment of ultimate good.[16]

And:

The Tao may never be left, even for a second. Anything that could be left would not be the true Tao.[17]

Mencius said that he nourished his vast, flowing ch'i. That is correct, but then always keep it in the tan-t'ien.

This is my humble experience. If you practice these points with perseverance you will discover taichi to be the world's finest exercise, and health and longevity to be simple affairs.

Discussions

CAN TAICHI REALLY be learned solely from a book, without any teacher? An excellent question! The ancients believed firmly in an oral tradition and the absolute necessity of personal instruction. So though taichi self-cultivation is an arduous task, success is certainly possible if your goal is health and vitality. If taichi's self-defense applications interest you, however, you must take every opportunity to practice push-hands with others. In this area, each student exhibits a different level of technical prowess—from the brutish to the sensitive—all based upon their intellectual makeup or characteristic proclivities. The letters I have received from rural students asking for advice fall like snowflakes around my desk. I cannot answer each one individually and so I borrowed some time from my busy schedule to write this book and fulfill their hopes. I had no other choice, for in my fervent wish to help others, every option had to be evaluated regardless of the difficulties involved.

One day in 1936, an old friend visited me in Nanking and asked for some taichi lessons to regain his health. I selected five postures: Ward-Off, Roll-Back, Press, Push, and Single Whip, and taught him how to practice. We parted soon afterward and did not meet again until the summer of 1939 in Szechuan. He then performed the entire form for me and asked for corrections. I asked him the name of his teacher. He laughed and said,

"You." I reminded him that I had taught him only five postures, not the full 120 posture form. He replied, "After we parted, I bought a copy of Yang Ch'eng-fu's *Uniting Form with Application in Taichi* and taught myself the form." I was impressed by his ability to deduce the entire form from those few postures. The form postures in Yang's book are explained from a functional, combative perspective and are often quite confusing. I employ quite a different format in my *New Method* work, and with careful practice, the reader should encounter no problems.

From my forty years of taichi practice, I have found that the defining aphorism in learning is this: What is most vital is least confusing. When I was studying with Yang Ch'eng-fu, he taught, scolded, and advised all with the same word: *relax.* In my first two years of study he repeated this word so many thousands of times that my head felt as crammed as an overstuffed basket. My incompetence disturbed me and I wondered how I arrived at such a sorrowful state. Then one night, I dreamt that both my arms were severed from my body. The next morning I applied this sensation to my taichi and achieved a new level of relaxation. My sinews and vessels felt connected to my arms with no more strength than rubber bands connect a baby doll's arms—they could maneuver freely and unobstructed. Only when my two arms felt almost disconnected could I sense true relaxation. All of my senior classmates were amazed at my sudden improvement, and after repeated questioning, discovered that I was really relaxed. I had leapt forward a thousand miles in a single day. I understand now the love and hope my teacher had for me. His vital teaching was not confusing; I was too ignorant to understand. Trust relaxation implicitly and practice it with devotion. Though I understood the marvels of relaxation over thirty years ago—even publishing them in my *Thirteen Treatises*—few people believe I divulged the true secret of taichi, and so, few understand true relaxation. Pay close attention as I once again outline the important aspects of relaxation.

Taichi was created to improve health and longevity, and its efficacy outweighs any doubts surrounding its historical origins. I would not practice an ineffectual exercise even if it was conclusively attributable to the Yellow Emperor or Lao Tzu. It is pointless to doubt that the Immortal Chang San-feng created taichi. Taichi was considered one of the noblest arts taught at Wutang, the "Forest of Martial Arts." Most of the martial training at the time involved boxing, and all were passed down from father to son either orally or through secret manuals. Historical research into taichi's origins based solely on written records or physical evidence is laughable.

Chang San-feng's sobriquet was "Seven Needle." Other men had similar given names, so we must be careful to write his name using the correct Chinese character. I have carefully pondered his *Discourse on Taichi* and find it to be a slice of pure, spiritual ch'i produced from a natural spontaneity. I do not know who else could have produced such a work. (The original footnote to the classic does mention his name as the author.) Chang was able to find practical applications from profound principles of wisdom embodied in classical literature. For example, Lao Tzu's principle stating that, "If you want to take, you must first give" was elaborated into taichi language by Chang, "If we wish to lift something, first push down. The root will then break naturally and the opponent will be thrown out." This is in part why taichi is the most ingenious martial art ever created, and why San-feng's achievement has never been equaled. Those who doubt his talents only serve to prove Lao Tzu's statement, "A lowly scholar laughs at the Tao. If he did not, it would not be the Tao."[18]

Chang San-feng is revered both as the founder of the Wutang School and the internal art of taichi. Bodhidharma established the external art of Shaolin. There is some confusion on how to distinguish an internal system from an external system. Chang San-feng imprinted the wisdom he culled from Huang-Lao cults into taichi; his system is internal because it originates from within the Chinese mind. (Huang, or the Yellow Emperor, is the legendary father of the Chinese race; Lao Tzu promoted his art of teaching.) Bodhidharma was a Buddhist whose teachings entered China from India; his system is external because it originated from a foreign land.

Moreover, taichi stresses sinking your ch'i to the tan-t'ien, extrapolated from Lao Tzu's concept of concentrating your ch'i to become soft and young. The Taoist phrase, "The waterwheel spins backward," depicts the flow of chi as it travels up your spinal *T'u* Meridian, passing first through your *wei-lu*, then the Jade Pillow, and on up to your ni-wan point. This process is called "Opening the Three Gates" and is explained in the Taichi Classics: "When your *wei-lu* is centered and straight, your spirit can rise to your headtop." Seminal energy is worked until it transmutes into ch'i; ch'i is worked until it transmutes into spirit—which probably proceeds from within the bones. Conversely, Bodhidharma's arts as explained in his *Sinew Changing* and *Marrow Cleansing* classics do develop ch'i, but the ch'i is allowed to proceed along its natural course up your frontal *Jen* Meridian to your face. The ch'i hardens because it follows your sinews and vessels without changing into spirit—attributes of an external system.

Taichi places a high emphasis on ch'i, as seen from the following examples taken from the classics:

Sink your chi to the tan-t'ien.

Move your ch'i with your mind, your body with ch'i.

Your ch'i must stick to your back whether pushing or pulling, advancing or retreating.

Your ch'i must be nourished without harm.

Arouse your ch'i.

Ch'i moves like a cart's axle; like a nine-curved string of pearls.

Advantages appear wherever ch'i goes.

Ch'i should fill your entire body without stagnating.

Your mind and ch'i are the prince, bones and muscles are vassals.

Collect your ch'i within.

These benefits come from applying concentrated ch'i. I will give a general outline on refining your ch'i and the steps that lead to its many benefits.

Refine your ch'i by first learning to sink it to the tan-t'ien, which is 1.3 inches beneath the navel—closer to the abdomen than the spine by a ratio of three to seven. Breathe in attentively and sink this ch'i slowly; abrupt breathing causes ch'i to rise. The four secret words for proper breathing are: fine, long, calm, and slow. Once you can do this remember to do it always and everywhere. Keeping both your mind and ch'i in the tan-t'ien directly nourishes it without harm. That taichi places attention on ch'i and not physique is seen in the phrase, "Your mind and ch'i are the prince, bone and muscle are vassals." At this level you have the basic skill to progress smoothly.

The first step in learning to move your ch'i is to make sure your mind moves your ch'i and ch'i moves your body. Arouse your ch'i and move it like a cart's axle; let it stick to your back as you push or pull, advance or retreat. When your ch'i can move through your body like a nine-curved string of pearls it brings advantages wherever it goes and fills your entire body without stagnating. When applying ch'i, the abdomen must be completely relaxed to allow it to spring forth. At its zenith, your ch'i sinks into the bones and collects in the spine. These are the benefits of concentrating your ch'i to become soft and young. When you understand how to refine your ch'i and transform it into spirit you can place your intention on essence and spirit, not merely on ch'i, because your movements stagnate when your intention is focused on ch'i. "Where there is ch'i there is no strength; where there is no ch'i there is pure hardness."[19] Such ch'i is transformed from essence ch'i and is one step removed from unrefined blood ch'i. Essence ch'i that transmutes into spirit produces divine strength, pure energy incomparable to ordinary ch'i. This level exhibits a technique that approaches the Tao. Never be satisfied with being merely an unbeatable hero.

Internal systems are those based on the wisdom of the Yellow Emperor and Lao Tzu. Nourishing ch'i and regulating breath are complicated subjects. The incipient movement of these two factors remain undetected and unmeasurable if weighed upon the scales of modern Western medicine, and relegates the student lacking a clear understanding of the *Classic on Internal Medicine* to a peripheral position. Western physicians recognize breath but not ch'i; they can see your diaphragm but not your tan-t'ien; they know how your muscles tighten and relax, bend and stretch, but not the underlying movement of your ch'i; they learn how to strengthen your skeletal bones and joints but not how to increase your essence ch'i to supplement marrow and precipitate internal transformations; they understand your nervous system and the movement of psychical energies but not the subtle marvels of your spiritual mind; they understand the circulatory system and cellular metabolism but not the system of mutual repletion and depletion in the Five Processes as applied to the Five Viscera or the ebb and flow of yin/yang. These examples are only the most commonly understood ones.

There are three distinctions of ch'i. The first is inside your body—blood ch'i; this is our foundational ch'i and it must be kept at thirty-seven degrees Celsius. The second form is outside your body—air ch'i; this is the stuff we breathe and it can be connected to the tan-t'ien, the so-called Sea of Ch'i, or Room of Stored Essence. Nourishing your ch'i by sinking your breath to the tan-t'ien warms your essence ch'i into the third form of ch'i—*yuan* ch'i. This ch'i connects the body's membranes and permeates the bones. I have discussed this in-depth in my *Thirteen Treatises*.

The diaphragm is the pivot and bowspring for ch'i. There are 656 separate muscle expansions or contractions in your body. To disregard ch'i as the impetus for your movements is to characterize your body as little more than one large, complicated, automated machine. Your bones and joints may be exercised till strong, but without marrow to fill them, they would dry out and become brittle. Nerves produce sensations and psychical energies move about, but without the spiritual mind to both issue and sort the sensations, both physical and mental sensations would retard. If blood circulation or cellular metabolism did not follow their proper repletion and depletion according to the Five [Processes and their respective—mh] Viscera, although blood cells are distinguished into red or white, they would not be in correspondence with the yin/yang distinction. Any Western physician would be confused when reading these ideas, yet it is rare to find one who has retained his scientific curiosity of the unknown. I invite all scientists to study the effects of taichi's substance and application. Its principle pervades every aspect of life—whether internal or external, superficial or refined—and its benefits are easily seen. They will understand that the mystery surrounding ch'i transformation in the arts of self-defense and health are in complete accord with scientific principles. Any martial art or sport that ignores this and searches for something else will be limited to a fraction of its potential.[20]

The Important Points
of Self-Cultivation

WHEN YOU PRACTICE the form try to remember: *All parts either move together or rest together; support your entire body upon a single leg.* Let your waist guide your movements. Every part of your body must follow your waist, from the bottom of your feet to the top of your head—even your vision. "Do not move your hands" means to not move your hands or feet independent of the waist.

When your wei-lu is centered and straight, your spirit can rise to your headtop. The entire body should be light and nimble. When your wei-lu is malaligned your spirit cannot rise. Carry your head atop your body with the same sensation as if you were suspended by your braided hair from the rafters above. If your head bobs and swings you may practice taichi fruitlessly for thirty years.

Every point throughout your body has the potential for full and empty. Without full and empty there would be no yin or yang; without yin or yang there is no taichi. The yin/yang distinction in your hands or legs is expressed physically as full and empty. The crisscross pathway of the nervous system requires you to coordinate your left arm with the right leg and your right arm with the left leg. Moreover, every part of your body—whether it lies to the left, right, above, or below—must be distinguished into full and empty; every point possesses this dual potential.

You must support your entire weight by a single, full leg which is properly rooted. If both legs use energy at the same time you are double-weighted. The double-weighted Horse-stance Posture in shaolin is taichi's most forbidden fault!

Every joint in your body must be strung together. This allows ch'i to pass smoothly through your body and benefits both form and application. Issuing energy and uprooting your opponent especially requires a unified form if the fulcrum principle is ever to be employed properly. A malaligned body simply scatters your energy and retards your mental directives.

Arouse your ch'i and interact. This means to invigorate your ch'i in the tan-t'ien and interact it with air ch'i. In the chapter entitled "Swimming on Land" from my *Thirteen Treatises,* I spoke of envisioning the air we breathe to be like water. Water can swirl and accumulate into a powerful force—its insubstantiality waxes into substantiality. Conversely, if we can imagine a powerful opponent as inconsequential as a puff of air, we can make his substantiality wane into insubstantiality.

When essence and spirit are strengthened internally, externally your body appears comfortable. This expresses taichi's ability to unify inner substantive strength with outer functional imperturbability. "Calm before an avalanche, composed beside a beast."[21] This is why Mencius said he cultivated his vast, flowing ch'i.

Long Boxing is like the slow continuous movement of great rivers and seas. The original thirteen postures of taichi were called "Long Boxing" because its ceaseless movement was coupled with momentum. All movement originates from an activating impetus. Thus, a train, plane, or car can move only after an impetus is conveyed from the engine to the wheels. Momentum, the surplus energy of all movement, was expressed in the *I Ching,* "The firm and soft touch each other; the eight trigrams displace one another."[22] This means that when A displaces B, B moves by momentum. All movement produces momentum that can, if unimpeded, provide additional impetus for further movement. These two forces can circle back and forth indefinitely. The original thirteen postures of taichi were described as Long Boxing because of the emphasis on continuity, not length of form. Even if the taichi form extended to ten thousand postures we could not call it Long Boxing unless we performed it as one continuous movement.

The only true secret in taichi is the phrase: *Your mind is the commander.* Your mind moves your chi, and ch'i transports your body through an initial impetus. Your hands and feet never move independently but wait until your waist clearly receives the mental command—then they follow the waist. So when we read that in taichi the hands should not move, this includes the feet. Also, remember to move as if every part is strung together on a single thread.

Translator's Notes

1. Confucius' statement was, "the Necessary Desires of man are; food, drink, and sexual pleasures." See James Legge, *The Book of Rites* (New York: University Books, 1967), p. 380.

2. *The Yellow Emperor's Classic on Internal Medicine (Huang-ti Nei-ching),* chapters 1:3, and 1:2.

3. Ibid., 69:1.

4. *Analects,* 13:22. The term *wu-i* refers to a healing sorceress. Legge's "wizard or a doctor" is wrong on two points: wrong grammar and wrong gender. See James Legge, vol. I, *The Chinese Classics* (Hong Kong: Hong Kong University Press, 1960), p. 272. The Shuo Wen describes the word *wu* as "A woman capable of serving the formless ones; by dancing she induces the spirits to descend." Recent scholarship has shown that in Shang times the sorceress played an important part of state-sponsored ceremonies. By later Chou times the sorceress had become incompatible with the emerging humanistic trends in Chinese thought, as evident from Confucius' characterization of her unorthodoxology. Thereupon, they drifted into the alternative, heterodoxical folk religions and healing arts, where they remain today. Nor can we employ the word "shaman," as Arthur Waley does in his translations. Mircea Eliade, the foremost authority on shamanism, dismisses spiritual possession where a spirit descends into the participant as an inferior form of shamanism. Shamanistic ecstasy, according to Eliade, is much more than mere spiritual possession. See Mircea Eliade, *Shamanism,* Bolligen Series 76 (New York: Pantheon Books, 1964), p. 23.

5. *Tao Teh Ching,* #22.

6. Cheng Man-ch'ing believed he had a close affinity to this T'ang poet, painter, and calligrapher named K'uan Wen. His friends often brought up the similarities between the two men and their lives. Late in life, the Professor even had a sobriquet seal carved, "The one born twelve hundred years after K'uan Wen."

7. *I Ching*, "*Hsi Tzu Ch'uan*," chapter A1:7.

8. The compound *chueh hsueh* means either "lost art" or "unparalled learning." Wile, in his *Advanced Form*, 1985, p. 29, prefers the former interpretation. However, given the explosion of enthusiasm for taichi that occurred in the twenties and thirties, I find that position indefensible.

9. *Analects*, 13:17.

10. The first line is from Han Yu's essay, "Encouraging Study" (*Chin-hsueh Chieh*); the latter is from Tu Mu's Preface to his edition of the *Tso Commentary to the Spring and Autumn Annals*. In no translation of this essay, either from Cheng's own disciples or from Wile, have these quotes been properly sourced and attributed.

11. I interpret *chi* as "proper" and not as a nominative pronoun. Examples of such an interpretation are too numerous to cite.

12. Hun Yuan is an ancient idea denoting the state of existance prior to the yin and yang division, primal confusion. Man is the "post" for connecting the two, eliminating their differentiation.

13. *Tao Teh Ching*, #50.

14. Cheng's original text mistakenly attributes the Hsun quote to Mencius.

15. The Three Potentials *(San Ts'ai)* originate from the *I Ching* and refers to the three individual lines of a trigram and represent heaven, earth, and man. When the trigrams have been doubled to a hexagram, all lines have reached their zenith and are then called the Three Extremes *(San Chi)*.

16. Truncated quote from the *Great Learning*, 2:1.

17. *Doctrine of the Mean* (*Chung Yung*), 1.

18. *Tao Teh Ching*, #41.

19. The contradictory expression, "no-ch'i," is a common Taoist metaphor which, as in "nonaction," does not refer to the absence of ch'i, but rather its ubiquity resulting from nonpartial, nondeliberate attentiveness. For the Professor's own thoughts on the matter, refer to Cheng's Introduction to Yang Ch'eng-fu's book, *Uniting Form with Application in Taichi*, translated in my *Cheng Man-ch'ing: Master of Five Excellences*, (Berkeley: Frog Ltd. 1995).

20. In the *Advanced Form* 1985, p.17, Wile omits these last two sentences.

21. Here again, as in footnote 14, Cheng quotes Hsun Shih's "The Art of the Heart/Mind" *(Hsin Shu)* and follows it with the Mencius quote. This second reference to the Hsun quote followed directly by Mencius's *vade mecum* proves that the Professor did in fact confuse the two. Modern indexes to both works should quickly put to rest any doubt of the Hsun quote coming from Mencius, a point overlooked in Wile, 1985, p. 25.

22. *I Ching*, "*Hsi Tzu Ch'uan*," A1:2.

The Simplified
Thirty-Seven Posture Form,
with Explanation
and Illustrations

Foot Diagrams

The Seven Variations
of Weight Posture Are:

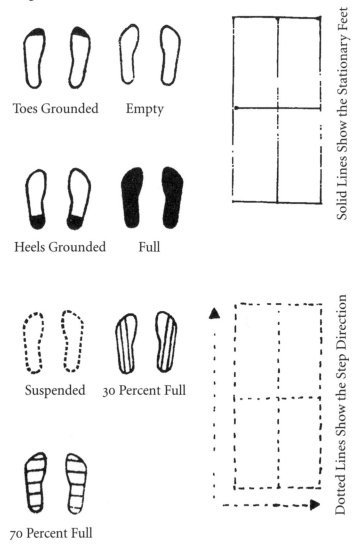

Toes Grounded   Empty

Heels Grounded   Full

Suspended   30 Percent Full

70 Percent Full

Solid Lines Show the Stationary Feet

Dotted Lines Show the Step Direction

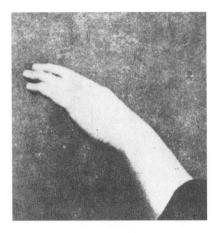

The Open Hand: Traditionally called the "Beautiful Lady's Hand," the backside tendons must never be stretched, and the wrist extends naturally.

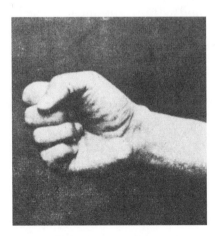

The Fist: Similar to an ordinary clenched fist, it appears tense but internally it remains relaxed. The top of the wrist extends naturally without bending.

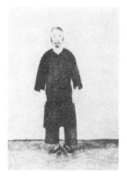 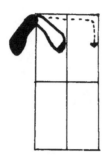 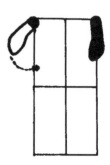

PICTURE 1   FOOT DIAGRAM 1   FOOT DIAGRAM 2

One: Preparation Posture

This is the standing meditative posture that cultivates undifferentiated ch'i (*yuan ch'i*). Starting from a balanced stance, undivided into full and empty, shift your weight onto your right leg, bend the knee, and sit fully into the leg. The left leg becomes empty and the heel rises. At the same time, both forearms rise about two to three inches, slightly arching the arms. Connect the ch'i up from the filling right leg through to the *lao-kung* point in the left palm's center. Such correspondence connects the interlaced pathway of nerves—see Picture 1, Foot Diagram 1.

Proceeding on, take one step to the left with your left foot and shift onto it—as in Foot Diagram 2. The tip of the right foot pivots parallel with the left foot, about a shoulder width apart. Stand up slowly until both legs are equally filled, knees neither bent nor locked.

This posture represents taichi before it has separated into yin and yang. As seen in Posture One, Foot Diagram 3, keep the elbows bent and the wrists arched slightly toward the front. The fingers point somewhat forward and are neither spread unevenly apart nor closed tightly.

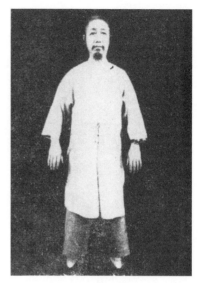

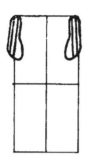

FOOT DIAGRAM 3

Posture One

Keep your head straight and erect. Your eyes gaze forward but you should look within and listen only to your breathing. Keep your mouth closed, lips together, with your tongue touching the roof of the palate. Sink the shoulders, drop the elbows, and empty the chest, because this helps the ch'i sink to the tan-t'ien. Breath fine, long, calm, and slow. Relax and open both internally and externally. Relax the entire body downward, remain completely natural. Connect the mind to the ch'i, from the wei-lu to the headtop. Work on unifying the external with the internal. Form and function arise from this posture—do not neglect it! You must understand this first posture clearly.

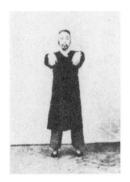
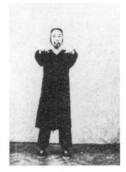
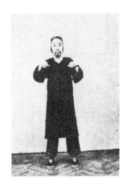

PICTURE 2   PICTURE 3   PICTURE 4

Two: Beginning Posture

This posture represents the metaphysical taichi producing the Two Aspects, yin and yang. Yin represents form—it lies below and is quiet; yang represents ch'i—it lies above as heaven and is light and pure, ascending movement.

At the beginning, move the ch'i with the mind and sink it to the tan-t'ien. Once the ch'i is abundant, the two arms follow the ch'i and rise; this is called "moving the ch'i with the mind." Your body expands when you breathe in, and contracts when you breathe out—the exhalation precipitates your arms descent. From here on, move your body with ch'i alone. Every movement in taichi, whether rising, falling, gathering, or expelling, is based on this initial move.

This first posture is designed to relax your wrists. The wrists change in six distinctive positions. From Standing Erect to the Preparation Posture is the first change. In the Beginning Posture, the arms float up with the wrists leading the way, fingers hanging down; this is the second change—see Picture 2. When the wrists reach shoulder height, direct your ch'i to extend the fingers. The hands' tendons and vessels must not be taunt; this is the third change—see Picture 3. Next, draw your arms back, folding the wrists and elbows in front of the chest; this is the

36

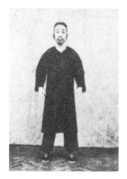 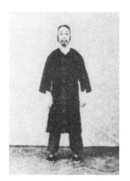

PICTURE 5   PICTURE 6

fourth change—see Picture 4. Drop the arms so the wrists appear as if they were sinking in water while the fingers remain at the surface; this is the fifth change—see Picture 5. Drop the arms to the side of the hip joints, their original position; this is the sixth change—see Picture 6.

As you can see, the Beginning Posture exercises the wrists. Relaxing these opens the first, pivotal posture in taichi. From here on, extend the ch'i through the wrists out to the fingers and maintain the Beautiful Lady's Hand. Pay careful attention to my explanations, for I will not repeat many ideas.

Three: Grasp the Sparrow's Tail, Left Ward-Off

Grasp the Sparrow's Tail is an ancient dance similar to "Grasp the Ox's Tail." But here it is employed as a generic term applied to the four movements Ward-Off, Roll-Back, Press, and Push—the basic postures of Push Hands. Push Hands is a two-man form that emphasizes sticking and adhering to an opponent. Both partners alternately perform these four basic moves, circling back and forth, trying not to disconnect nor resist. A player's arms are compared to a sparrow's tail, which each opponent tries to grasp. Push Hands develops a sensitivity for interpret-

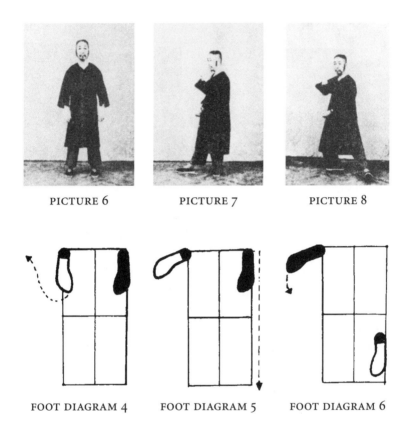

PICTURE 6   PICTURE 7   PICTURE 8

FOOT DIAGRAM 4   FOOT DIAGRAM 5   FOOT DIAGRAM 6

ing energy and is indicative of this exercise's potential for high levels of awareness.

Left Ward-Off begins where Beginning Posture concludes. Shift onto the left leg, bend the knee and sit fully on it; the left leg is full and the right is empty—see Picture 6, Foot Diagram 4. Turn the waist/hip joint right. Raise the tip of the right foot and, following the waist, pivot right. At the same time, the right arm, which followed beside the right waist, rises and turns right, level with the armpit, palm down. Simultaneously, the left hand turns to the right until it is level with the right hip joint, palm up. The two hands look as if they are holding something—as in Picture 7, Foot Diagram 5.

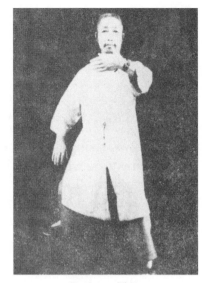

Posture Two

Sit fully on your right leg, raise your left heel, and turn to the front left side. Step directly forward with your left foot, as shown by the directional arrows, heel first, toes slightly raised—as in Picture 8, Foot Diagram 6.

Shift gradually onto the left leg until full. At the same time, the left hand rises, following the waist/hip joint, and performs a Ward-Off at chest level, palm in, and elbow hanging slightly down. Simultaneously, drop the right hand to the right side of the hip, slightly curved, corresponding to the left leg's full strength. Pivot the right toes in forty-five degrees—see Posture Two, Foot Diagram 7.

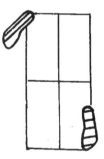

FOOT DIAGRAM 7

The important points to remember about this posture are: the left and right hip joints must be centered and straight; the left knee should be directly over the toes, never beyond; the right knee is slightly bent; draw in the wei-lu till it is centered and straight—enabling the spirit to connect through to the head. The front leg is 70 percent full and planted directly into the ground, the rear leg is 30 percent full and contains the active strength that presses forward.

Three: Grasp the Sparrow's Tail, Right Ward-Off

Continuing on, relax the right waist/hip joint and shift forward completely onto the front leg. Lift the right heel and turn it slightly to the left following the waist. Turn the right hand over to the left side, palm up, next to the left hip joint. The left palm also turns over, and the two hands appear to be holding something—see Picture 9, Foot Diagram 8.

Now raise the right foot and place the heel down where the toes were. Shift onto it until full, while the left leg changes to empty, and the toes turn in forty-five degrees to the front. Simultaneously, raise the right elbow and perform a Ward-Off at chest level, palm in. Straighten the left open hand and push forward following the waist, stopping about six inches from the right hand, midway between the chest and the right hand—see Posture Three, Foot Diagram 9.

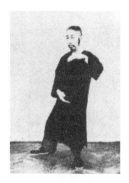

PICTURE 9

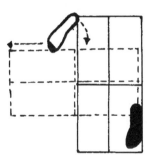

FOOT DIAGRAM 8

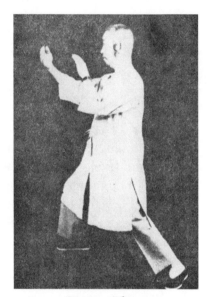

Posture Three

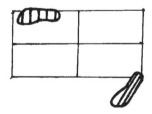

FOOT DIAGRAM 9

Four: Grasp the Sparrow's Tail, Roll-Back

Next, turn the left waist/hip joint slightly to the right-front corner, placing the weight entirely on the right leg. The two elbows momentate [move with momentum — mh] slightly forward — as in Picture 10, Foot Diagram 10. Relax the waist, turn, and shift back fully onto the left leg. Keep the right elbow and wrist erect, the right palm facing left. Turn over the left wrist following the waist, palm up, and place it beside the right elbow — see Posture Four, Foot Diagram 11.

Turn the waist as far as possible to the left rear. Following this movement, the two arms momentate to the left rear side, the feet remain fixed — as in Picture 11.

There are two points to remember in this posture. First, your eyesight should follow your head as it turns, looking directly forward and level — when the waist stops, maintain careful attention in that direction. Second, the hands must not only move with the waist, they rest when it rests. The excess energy of any movement is called momentum. Before this momentum dissipates, direct it toward the next movement. The true key to successful taichi is channeling the momentum of any movement into the next posture. Apply your energy cyclically from movement to momentum, and back to movement. The slightest break between the two forces results in discontinuity. I hope the reader will pay close attention to this, as I will not repeat it.

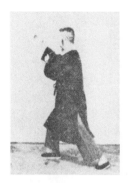

PICTURE 10

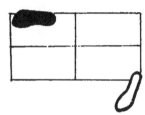

FOOT DIAGRAM 10

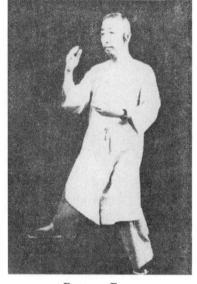

Posture Four

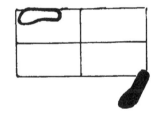

FOOT DIAGRAM 11

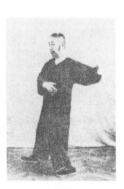

PICTURE 11

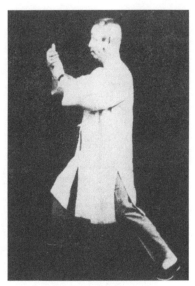

Posture Five

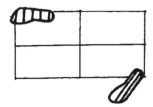

Five: Grasp the Sparrow's Tail, Press

When the arms' momentum is almost concluded, the right knee begins to return forward as you bend it slightly and sit fully on it. The waist/hip joint turns to the right front, and the two arms follow this and pull forward, momentating up. The right arm is even with the chest, as in Right Ward-Off. The full energy of the left hand corresponds with the full right leg—ch'i connects the two. Press forward following the waist, the open left hand adhering to the inner right wrist—see Posture Five, Foot Diagram 12.

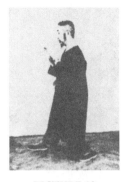

PICTURE 12

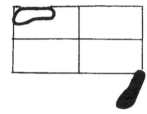

FOOT DIAGRAM 13

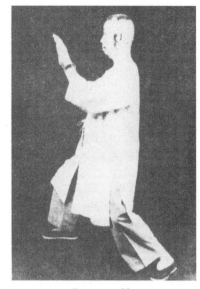

Posture Six

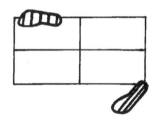

FOOT DIAGRAM 14

Six: Grasp the Sparrow's Tail, Push

Shift onto the left leg, bend the knee, and sit fully on it. At the same time, the two arms follow the waist and momentate back near the short ribs, palms forward—as in Picture 12, Foot Diagram 13. Straighten the left leg to the front, bend the right knee, and sit fully on it. Simultaneously, the two hands push straight forward—see Posture Six, Foot Diagram 14. Make sure all hand movement follows the movement and momentum of the waist—nothing moves independently. Remember this always!

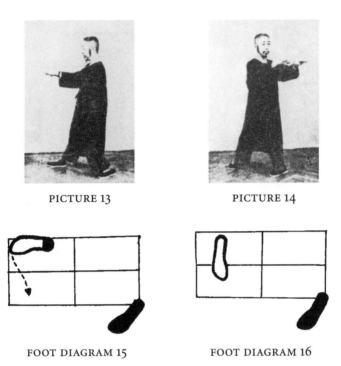

PICTURE 13   PICTURE 14

FOOT DIAGRAM 15   FOOT DIAGRAM 16

Seven: Single Whip

Shift back onto the left leg, bend the knee, and sit fully into it. At the same time, the two arms follow the waist and drop to chest level, palm down—as in Picture 13, Foot Diagram 15.

Turn the waist to the left, raise the tip of the right foot, and completely follow the waist as it turns. The two arms follow the waist and momentate to the left rear corner. When you can turn no further, there is a slight "settling down-rising up" movement—see Picture 14, Foot Diagram 16.

Bend the right knee and sit fully on the right leg. The two arms follow the waist and momentate in, the right hand changing to a hanging hand next to the right armpit. The left hand assists beneath the right elbow and armpit, palm up. The right

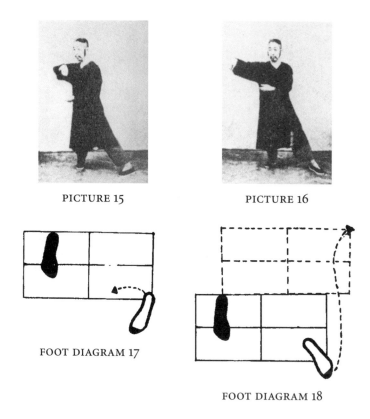

PICTURE 15   PICTURE 16

FOOT DIAGRAM 17

FOOT DIAGRAM 18

waist/hip joint sinks slightly—as in Picture 15, Foot Diagram 17.

The right wrist and hanging hand follow the waist and extend to the right-front corner. Raise the left hand up to the right short rib area. Note that the left heel is raised and follows the right hand's extension, turning to the right-front corner—as in Picture 16, Foot Diagram 18.

Raise the left leg and take a large step to the left front, heel first; step onto it slowly until full. Simultaneously, the left arm rises following the waist and assumes a preparatory, erect posture in front of the chest, the palm directly in front of your vision. The right wrist and hanging hand do not move and remain shoulder level; only the right elbow lowers slightly—as

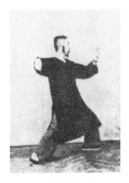

PICTURE 17

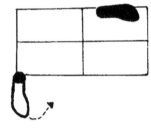

FOOT DIAGRAM 19

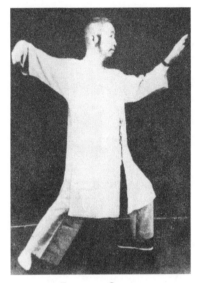

Posture Seven

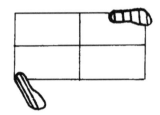

FOOT DIAGRAM 20

in Picture 17, Foot Diagram 19.

The right waist/hip joint turns forward until it is in line with the left, the right toes pivot in forty-five degrees. At the same time, turn the left hand over, palm out and shoulder level—see Posture Seven, Foot Diagram 20.

This posture is especially complicated, so be sure to remember all of the lessons I have already discussed. Keep your wei-lu centered and straight to allow spirit to connect through to your headtop, hold the head erect and balanced, and sink the ch'i to the tan-t'ien. All of these principles must be followed at every level. Move the body and limbs solely by following the waist, because nothing moves independently—remember this! The Single Whip encompasses one hundred eighty degrees, passes through three directions, and contains many stages and transitions—additional personal guidance is absolutely necessary for proper performance and understanding. After you have refined the basic movement, try to complete the move in a single breath, a unified ch'i—one long flowing movement.

The Single Whip is taichi's most expansive posture and is used as a meditative posture that cultivates extension. With careful practice you should master it.

Eight: Lift Hands

As you sit fully on your left leg, your right leg changes to empty—see Foot Diagram 21. The right heel rises and turns toward the left, following the waist. As the same time the right hanging hand opens, relaxes, and sinks; the left hand also relaxes, sinks, and turns so that the palm is facing somewhat forward, opposite the right palm—as in Picture 18, Foot Diagram 22.

Raise the right leg to the front right side, heel touching the ground. The two feet form the letter "L". The two arms follow the waist and come together, palms in, left palm opposite right elbow—see Posture Eight, Foot Diagram 23.

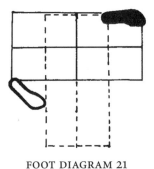

FOOT DIAGRAM 21

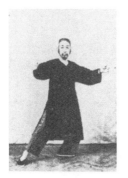

PICTURE 18

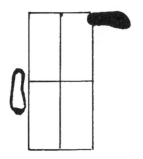

FOOT DIAGRAM 22

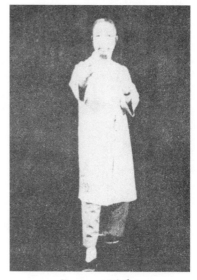

Posture Eight

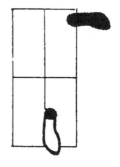

FOOT DIAGRAM 23

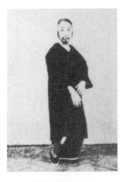

PICTURE 19

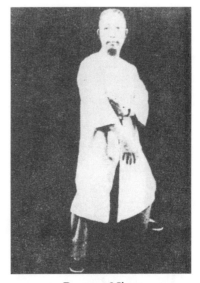

Posture Nine

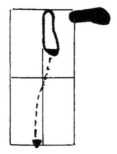

FOOT DIAGRAM 24

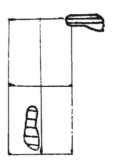

FOOT DIAGRAM 25

Nine: Shoulder Strike

While still on your left leg, drop the right arm and leg back in toward the body following the waist. The left arm follows and comes to rest by the left side of the hip joint—as in Picture 19, Foot Diagram 24.

The right leg steps directly forward, following the directional arrow, shifting slowly until full. The right elbow bends, palm in, so that the arm resembles a bow. The left hand assists near the inner right elbow—see Posture Nine, Foot Diagram 25.

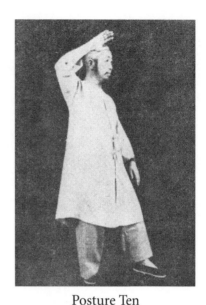

Posture Ten

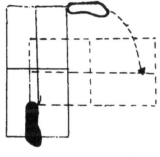

FOOT DIAGRAM 26

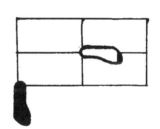

FOOT DIAGRAM 27

Ten: White Crane Spreads Its Wing

As you sit fully on the right leg, the left leg becomes empty—
as in Foot Diagram 26. Now raise the left foot and place the toes
off to the left-front side. At the same time, the right arm rises,
the open right hand moves up to protect the right side of the
forehead, and the palm faces the right-front corner. The left
hand turns and drops, brushing past the knee to protect the
groin, assisting next to the left hip joint—see Posture Ten, Foot
Diagram 27.

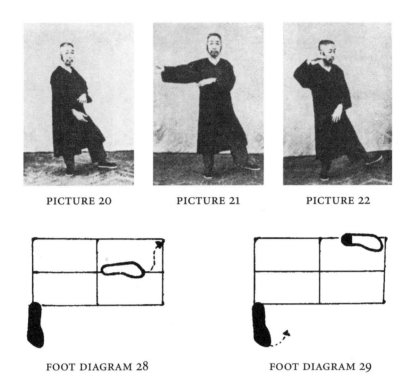

PICTURE 20   PICTURE 21   PICTURE 22

FOOT DIAGRAM 28   FOOT DIAGRAM 29

Eleven: Brush Left Knee, Twist Step

As you drop fully on the right leg, the left leg becomes empty. Drop the right arm following the waist, and place it next to the right leg. The left hand moves slightly to the right—as in Picture 20, Foot Diagram 28.

As the waist turns to the right rear, the two arms follow in momentum—see Picture 21; the feet remain stationary.

Lift the left leg and step to the front, heel first. The right arm follows the right rear turning of the waist and circles from bottom to top, returning to prepare the posture next to the right ear, palm down. The left arm momentates toward the right side, preparing for the posture next to the front right side of the crotch—as in Picture 22, Foot Diagram 29.

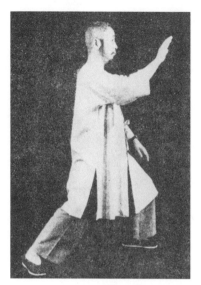

Posture Eleven

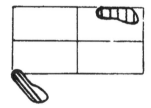

FOOT DIAGRAM 30

Shift slowly onto the left leg until full. The right open hand follows the waist and slices forward. Hang your elbows, sit on your wrist, and erect your open hand—follow the waist as you push forward. Simultaneously, the right toes pivot in forty-five degrees. The left hand protects the crotch by brushing over to the left knee, and is prepared to assist next to the left hip joint— see Posture Eleven, Foot Diagram 30.

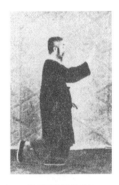

PICTURE 23

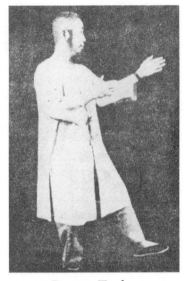

Posture Twelve

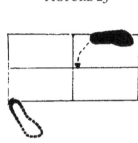

FOOT DIAGRAM 31

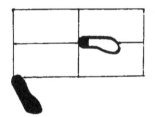

FOOT DIAGRAM 32

Twelve:
Strumming the Guitar

Shift fully on your left leg and raise the right toes slightly off the ground, the elbows extended slightly—as in Picture 23, Foot Diagram 31.

Drop the right leg back down and sit slowly on it until full. Draw the left foot about an inch, heel touching. At the same time, the right arm follows the waist and moves back in, stopping near the right short ribs, palm left. Raise the left hand, palm in, until it is opposite the right elbow. You appear to be holding a guitar—see Posture Twelve, Foot Diagram 32.

Brush Left Knee, Twist Step

Relax the right side of the waist, turn to the right rear, and shift completely onto the right leg. At the same time, the right arm follows the waist and circles up to prepare the posture near the right ear, palm down—as in Picture 24, Foot Diagram 33.

The left hand protects the crotch next to the left leg. Raise the right foot and take one half-step to the front left—as in Picture 25, Foot Diagram 34. Shift onto the left leg. The open right hand slices forward—be sure to hang the elbow, sit on the wrist, and erect the open hand, palm forward. The left hand brushes past the left knee and rests outside the left hip joint. The right

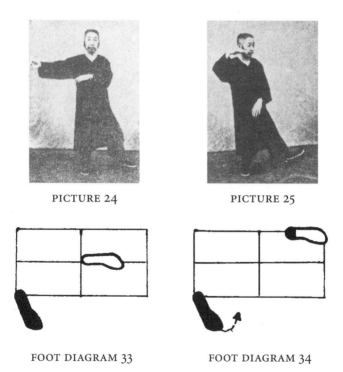

PICTURE 24   PICTURE 25

FOOT DIAGRAM 33   FOOT DIAGRAM 34

toes pivot forty-five degrees—as in Picture 26, Foot Diagram 35.

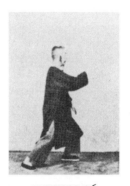

PICTURE 26

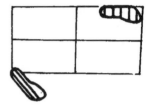

FOOT DIAGRAM 35

Thirteen: Step Forward, Block, Parry, Punch

Continuing on, shift fully onto the right, rear leg. The tip of the left foot pivots left forty-five degrees following the waist. At the same time, the right hand forms a fist and drops next to the inner left hip joint—as in Picture 27, Foot Diagram 36; also the accompanying Picture 28, taken from the opposite side. Sit gradually on the left leg until full. Raise the right foot and take one half-step toward the front right corner—as in Picture 29, Foot Diagram 37; also its accompanying Picture 30 taken from the opposite side.

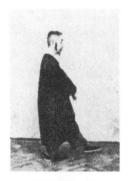

PICTURE 27

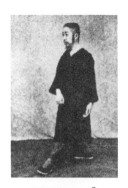

PICTURE 28

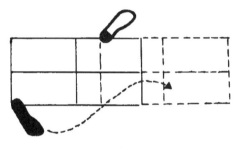

FOOT DIAGRAM 36

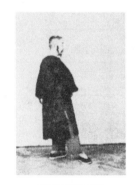

PICTURE 29

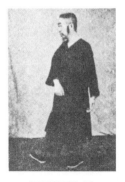

PICTURE 30

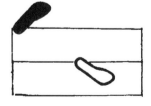

FOOT DIAGRAM 37

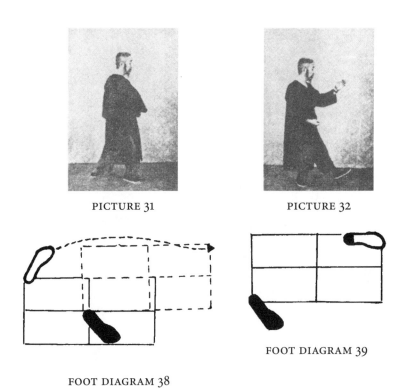

PICTURE 31   PICTURE 32

FOOT DIAGRAM 39

FOOT DIAGRAM 38

Shift fully onto the right leg, turning the waist/hip joint to the right—as in Picture 31, Foot Diagram 38. Take one large step to the left-front corner, heel first. The right fist simultaneously turns so that the Tiger Mouth [the circle created by the index finger and thumb in a fist posture—mh] faces right. Bring the right hand to rest next to the right short ribs. This movement is called Block. The left hand is open and stands erect like a cleaver, ready to intercept a frontal attack, so it is called Parry— see Picture 32, Foot Diagram 39.

Continuing on, shift fully onto the left leg. The right fist follows the waist and punches toward the front. The left open hand assists between the right wrist and elbow area. These three moves are called Block, Parry, and Punch — see Posture Thirteen, Foot Diagram 40.

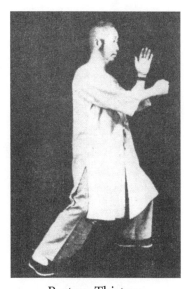

Posture Thirteen

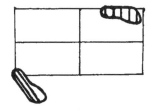

FOOT DIAGRAM 40

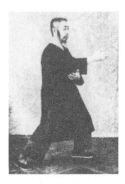

PICTURE 33

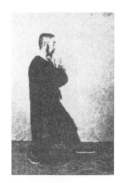

PICTURE 34

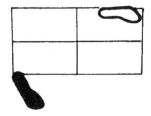

FOOT DIAGRAM 41

Fourteen: Apparently Sealing, Seemingly Closing

Proceeding on, the right hand changes to an open hand and follows the waist toward the left-front corner. The erect open hand turns over, palm up, and protects under the right elbow. The feet remain stationary—as in Picture 33.

Shift onto your right leg, relax the waist, bend the knee, and sit fully on the leg. The right hand moves to the left rear, and the left open hand sweeps the right elbow and moves up the arm until it meets up with the right wrist; the two wrists crisscross. This is called Apparently Sealing—see Picture 34, Foot Diagram 41.

Now shift onto the front left leg. The two hands turn around and separate, forming a Push posture. This is called Seemingly Closing—see Posture Fourteen, Foot Diagram 42.

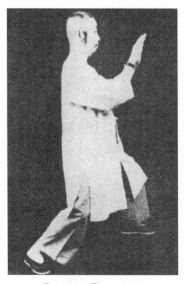

Posture Fourteen

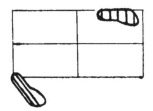

FOOT DIAGRAM 42

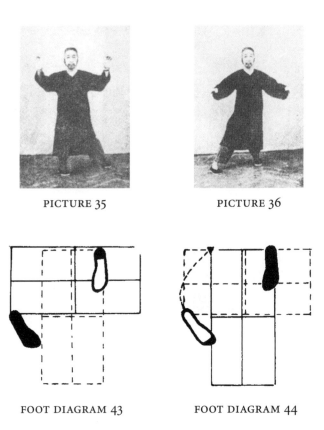

PICTURE 35   PICTURE 36

FOOT DIAGRAM 43   FOOT DIAGRAM 44

Fifteen: Cross Hands

Shift onto the right leg, bend the knee, and sit fully on the leg. The tip of the left foot rises and turns to the right front following the waist, turning until it is directly forward. The two arms follow the waist and gradually extend open — see Picture 35, Foot Diagram 43. As you shift onto the left leg, the right leg becomes empty. The two arms follow the waist and descend, palms down — see Picture 36, Foot Diagram 44.

Continuing on, bring the right foot back parallel with the left foot, as in the Beginning Posture. Gather the two arms together, intersecting at the wrists—left wrist above, right, below. This is called Cross Hands—see Posture Fifteen, Foot Diagram 45.

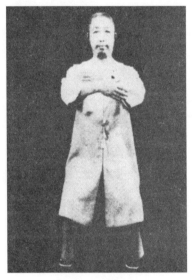

Posture Fifteen

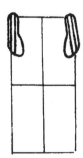

FOOT DIAGRAM 45

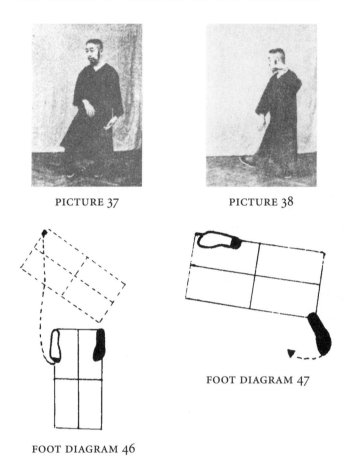

PICTURE 37

PICTURE 38

FOOT DIAGRAM 47

FOOT DIAGRAM 46

Sixteen: Embrace Tiger, Return to Mountain

Proceeding on, shift fully onto your left leg. Raise your right empty leg, heel first, and turn the waist/hip joint to the right rear corner. Simultaneously, the two arms relax and drop open, with the left elbow dropping first and moving the furthest—as in Picture 37, Foot Diagram 46.

Take one large step to the right rear. The left arm follows the waist and circles up to prepare the position next to the left ear. The right hand brushes the right knee and drops to the side—

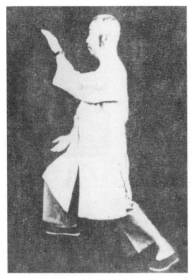

Posture Sixteen

as in Picture 38, Foot Diagram 47.

Shift slowly onto the right leg until full. At the same time, the left hand follows the left side of the waist/hip joint and slices forward, preparing the posture by sitting on the wrist and sinking the elbow. After the right hand has brushed the knee, it circles up to the side of the thigh, palm up. This is called Embrace Tiger — see Posture Sixteen, Foot Diagram 48.

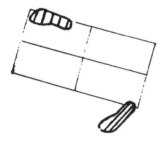

FOOT DIAGRAM 48

Note: Picture 39 shows the same posture from another angle.

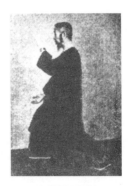

PICTURE 39

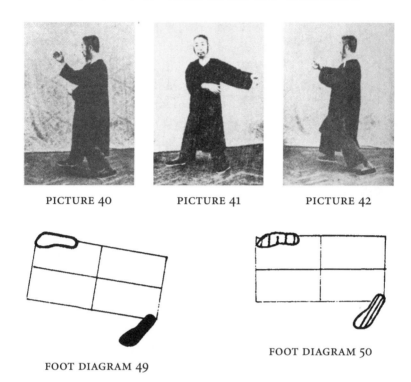

PICTURE 40   PICTURE 41   PICTURE 42

FOOT DIAGRAM 49

FOOT DIAGRAM 50

Grasping the Sparrow's Tail:
Ward-Off, Roll-Back, Press, Push

Continuing on, shift onto the left leg, bend the knee, and sit fully on it. At the same time, the right forearm turns over and up, palm facing left. The left wrist turns palm up, forming a Roll-Back—as in Picture 40, Foot Diagram 49.

The two arms follow the waist/hip joint and momentate to the left rear—as in Picture 41, the feet remain fixed. The two arms continue to follow the turning waist/hip joint. Shift onto the right leg, bend the knee, and sit fully on it. The right arm momentates into a Ward-Off posture, the left hand follows and adheres to the inside of the right wrist area. This is Press—see Picture 42, Foot Diagram 50.

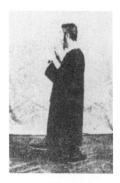

PICTURE 43

Shift onto the left rear leg, bend the knee, and sit fully on it. The two arms relax open and follow the waist/hip joint until they are in front of the chest, palms out—as in Picture 43, Foot Diagram 49. Continuing on, follow the waist/hip joint forward and shift onto the right leg, bend the knee, and sit fully on it. The two arms push forward. The back of the wrists should extend naturally, the waist and wei-lu must be vertical and aligned—as in Picture 44, Foot Diagram 50.

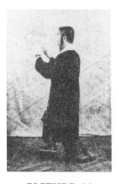

PICTURE 44

Diagonal Single Whip

The explanation of the Diagonal Single Whip is identical to the previous Single Whip.

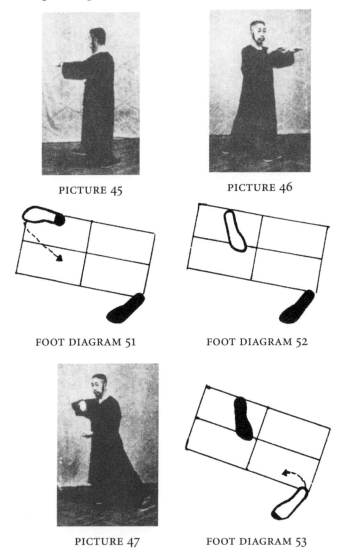

PICTURE 45

PICTURE 46

FOOT DIAGRAM 51

FOOT DIAGRAM 52

PICTURE 47

FOOT DIAGRAM 53

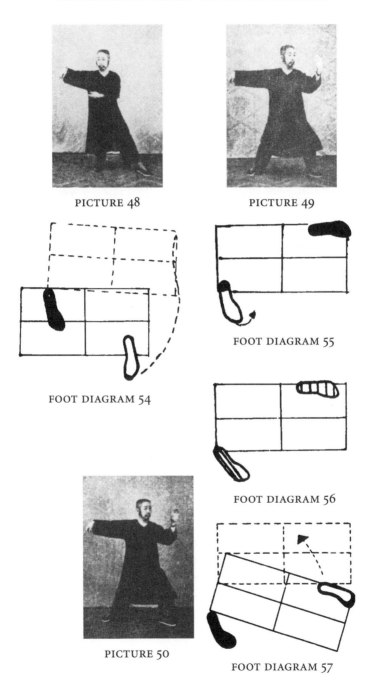

PICTURE 48

PICTURE 49

FOOT DIAGRAM 55

FOOT DIAGRAM 54

FOOT DIAGRAM 56

PICTURE 50

FOOT DIAGRAM 57

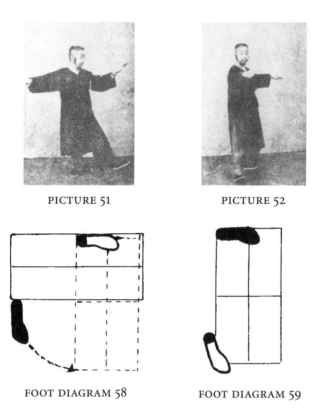

PICTURE 51   PICTURE 52

FOOT DIAGRAM 58   FOOT DIAGRAM 59

Seventeen: Rely on Fist below Elbow

Continuing on, shift onto the right leg, bend the knee, and sit fully on it. The right hanging hand relaxes open, the left open hands drops slightly. The left foot takes a step, heel first, toward the front-left side—as in Picture 51, Foot Diagram 58. Shift fully onto the left leg, then the right leg takes a step to the right front until the tip of the right foot is parallel with the heel of the left foot. The two arms turn, following the waist—as in Picture 52, Foot Diagram 59.

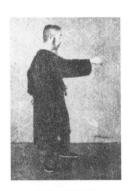

PICTURE 53

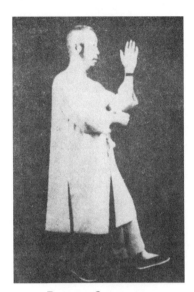

Posture Seventeen

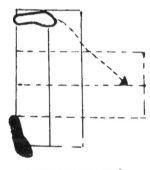

FOOT DIAGRAM 60

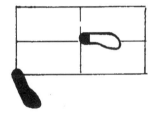

FOOT DIAGRAM 61

Continuing on, shift fully onto the right leg. The two arms continue to turn until the right arm is directly ahead, palm down, and the left arm is by the left side of the left hip joint, turning down in a small circle, palm facing the inner right side—see Picture 53, Foot Diagram 60.

Next, place the left foot directly in front, heel down. The left arm rises erect in front of the chest, palm right. Simultaneously, draw the right arm in, placing the fist under the elbow. This is called Rely on Fist below Elbow—see Posture Seventeen, Foot Diagram 61.

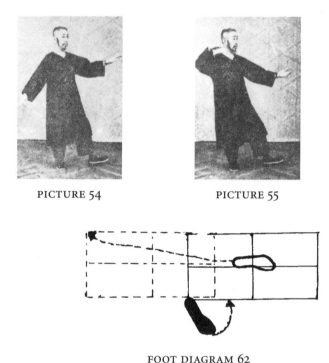

PICTURE 54 PICTURE 55

FOOT DIAGRAM 62

Eighteen: The Retreating Monkey

Relax and open the right hip joint to the right rear, while the right fist opens and follows the waist/hip joint, momentating to the right rear side. The erect left hand follows and descends, palm down—as in Picture 54, the feet remain stationary.

The right arm follows the waist and circles up until the over-turned hand comes to rest next to the right ear. Simultaneously, the left hand turns over, palm up—as in Picture 55, Foot Diagram 62.

Continuing on, step directly back with the left leg, toe first. Slowly bend the knee and sit fully on the leg. At the same time the right toes pivot to the left, bringing the two legs parallel and

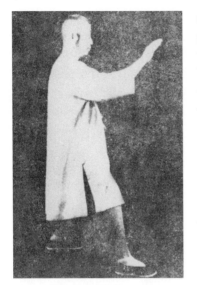

Posture Eighteen

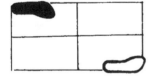

FOOT DIAGRAM 63

shoulder's width apart. The fingers of the right hand slice forward, and then are brought back to stand, following the waist. Draw the left hand back to the left hip joint, palm up— see Posture Eighteen, Foot Diagram 63.

Note: In the picture to the left, my left hand is blocked from view. Please refer to Posture Nineteen for the correct hand position when the right hand is down by the hip joint.

Now turn the waist/hip joint to the left rear. The right arm follows the waist and extends out about five to six inches. The left arm turns to the left rear and circles up next to the left ear, palm down. At the same time, the right wrist turns over, palm up— as in Picture 56, Foot Diagram 64.

Take one large step straight back with the right leg, toes first. Bend the knee and

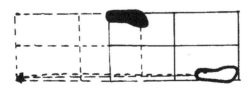

FOOT DIAGRAM 64

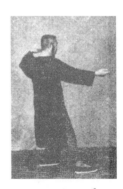

PICTURE 56

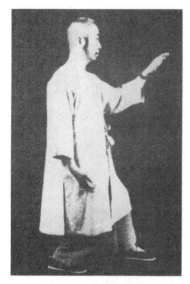

Posture Nineteen

sit fully on it. Draw the right arm back next to the right hip joint. At the same time, the left hand turns around and slices forward. Once the waist is stabilized, the left hand rests standing, gathering the position and setting the wrists—see Posture Nineteen, Foot Diagram 65.

Continuing on, turn the right waist/hip joint to the right rear. The right arm circles up and gathers the position next to the right ear, palm

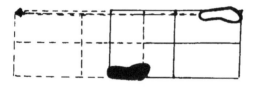

FOOT DIAGRAM 65

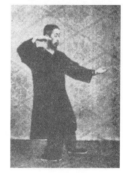

PICTURE 57

down. At the same time, the left elbow extends forward about five inches, then turns over together with the right hand, palm up—as in Picture 57, the feet remain stationary.

The left leg takes a large step straight back. The remaining movements are the same as above, so I will not repeat them here. This was the Left and Right forms for the Retreating Monkey—see Picture 57 and 58.

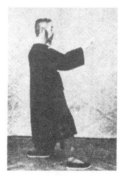

PICTURE 58

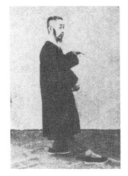

PICTURE 59

Twenty: Diagonal Flying Posture

Proceeding on, relax the right side of the waist and bring it together with the left hip joint. Drop the right hand down to the left hip joint, palm up. The left hand turns over and moves up under the right armpit—as in Picture 59, Foot Diagram 66.

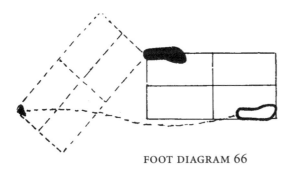

FOOT DIAGRAM 66

Turn to the right-rear corner and take a large step with the right leg, about one hundred seventy degrees. The left hand follows beside the waist. Raise the right hand to just below the left armpit—as in Picture 60, Foot Diagram 67.

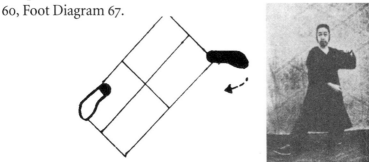

FOOT DIAGRAM 67

PICTURE 60

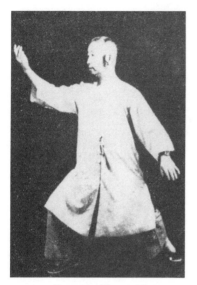

Posture Twenty

Proceeding on, shift onto the right leg, bend the knee, and sit fully on it. The right arm follows the waist and extends open, the left toes pivot in forty-five degrees. The left wrist descends down to the side of the left hip joint. This is the Diagonal Flying Posture—see Posture Twenty, Foot Diagram 68.

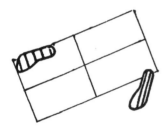

FOOT DIAGRAM 68

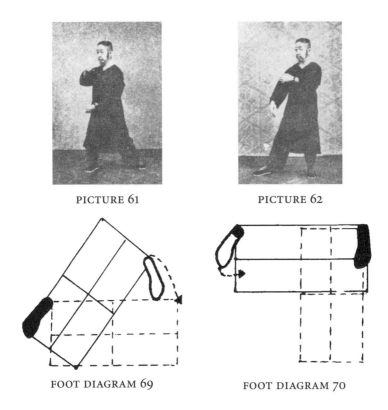

PICTURE 61   PICTURE 62

FOOT DIAGRAM 69   FOOT DIAGRAM 70

Twenty One: Cloud Hands

Continuing on, turn the waist/hip joint to the right and shift fully onto the right leg. The left hand follows and gathers in front of the right hip joint, palm up. Turn over the right wrist, palm down. Together, the two hands appear to be holding something. At the same time, take a small step with the left leg directly forward, bringing it parallel with the right leg—as in Picture 61, Foot Diagram 69.

Proceeding on, shift onto the left leg, bend the knee, and sit fully on it. At the same time, turn the waist/hip joint to the left front. Raise the left arm and perform a Ward-Off at chest level. Drop the right arm down beside the right hip joint, palm in— as in Picture 62, Foot Diagram 70.

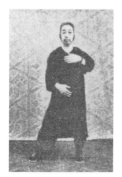

PICTURE 63

Continue turning the waist left, the two arms following opposite to each other; left on top, right on bottom. As the body turns forward, the right toes pivot to the front, bringing the two feet exactly parallel—as in Picture 63, Foot Diagram 71.

Continue to pivot to the left-front side, moving much like a grindstone turns. The two arms follow and appear to be holding something. The left arm turns until it is in front of the left side of the chest, and the right hand turns up and assists beneath the left lower abdomen. Raise the right foot and bring it parallel, one half-step away from the left foot, one shoulder width apart. This is

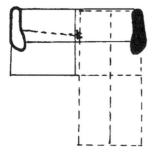

FOOT DIAGRAM 71

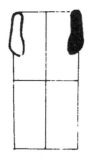

FOOT DIAGRAM 72

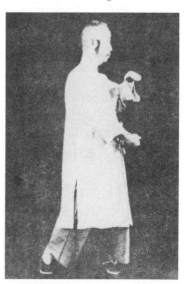

Posture Twenty-One

Cloud Hands—see Posture Twenty-One, Foot Diagram 72.

Proceeding on, shift onto the right leg, bend the knee, and sit fully on it. As the waist/hip joint begins to turn right, the two arms rise and descend as in the previous posture—see Picture 64, Foot Diagram 73.

Continue turning the waist to the right like a grindstone, exactly like the previous posture. As with Posture Twenty-Two, the feet remain stationary. After this posture is another Cloud Hands, Left, which is the same as before. First, take one half-step sideways to the left, about two shoulder widths apart. Sit fully on the left leg, then the two arms turn

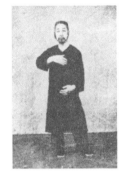

PICTURE 64

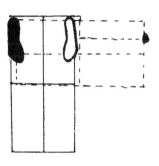

FOOT DIAGRAM 73

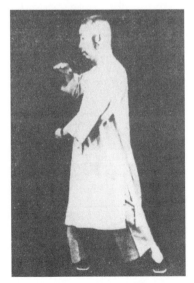

Posture Twenty-Two

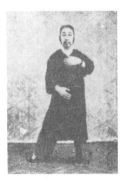

PICTURE 65

81

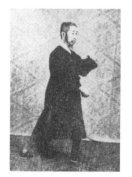

until directly in front—as in Picture 65. As you continue turning to the left, the two arms follow and appear to be holding something—as in Picture 66. After this posture there is one right and one left posture, before continuing on to Single Whip.

PICTURE 66

Twenty-Three: Squatting Single Whip

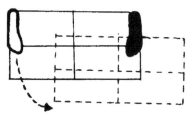

FOOT DIAGRAM 74

The right leg takes one half-step to the right front, as in Foot Diagram 74. Shift fully onto this leg, bend the knee, and sit on it. Raise the right hand, following the waist, to the right-front side, forming a hanging hand. Drop the left hand, palm over, to assist the right hanging hand under the right short ribs—as in Picture 67, Foot Diagram 75.

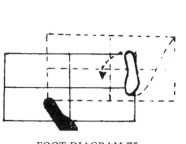

FOOT DIAGRAM 75

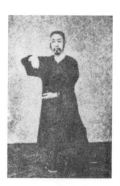

PICTURE 67

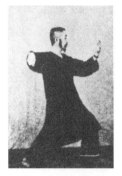

PICTURE 68

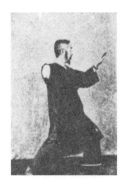

PICTURE 69

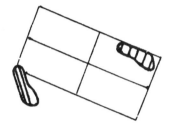

FOOT DIAGRAM 76

Continuing on, perform a Single Whip—as in Picture 68 and 69, Foot Diagram 76.

Next, sit fully onto the left leg as the right leg becomes empty. The right toes pivot right forty-five degrees as in Foot Diagram 77. As you shift onto the right leg, the left toes pivot in forty-five degrees. The left hand, which was pushing in front, draws back and drops down to the side of the crotch, fingers pointing down. The right hanging hand remains in position. The left toes now turn out

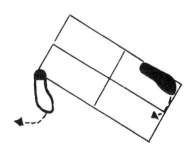

FOOT DIAGRAM 77

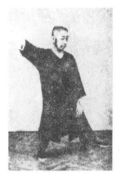

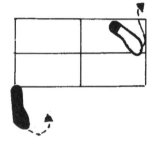

forty-five degrees—as in Picture 70, Foot Diagram 78.

Next, the waist, hip joint, and wei-lu all descend. The left hand creeps down the left leg, directly past the toes—as with Posture Twenty-Three, the feet remain stationary.

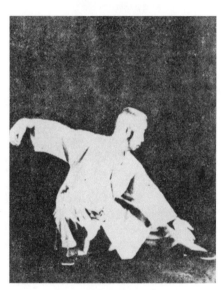

Posture Twenty-Three

Twenty-Four: Right Golden Chicken Stands on One Leg

Continuing on, pivot the left foot ninety degrees out toward the left-front corner. Shift onto the left leg, bend the knee, and sit fully on it. Simultaneously, the right foot pivots in forty-five degrees, and the heel rises off the ground. Relax, open the right hanging hand, and bring it next to the right hip joint—as in Picture 71, Foot Diagram 70.

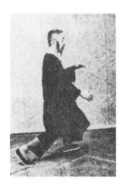

PICTURE 71

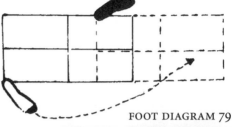

FOOT DIAGRAM 79

At the same time, the right leg follows the shifting and rises up to meet the right elbow. The right foot toes hang down, and the left hand descends to assist next to the left hip joint, palm down. This is Right Golden Chicken Stands on One Leg— see Posture Twenty-Four, Foot Diagram 80.

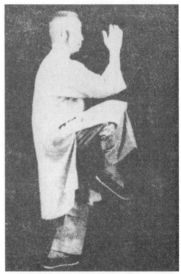

Posture Twenty-Four

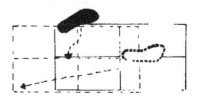

FOOT DIAGRAM 80

85

Twenty-Five: Left Golden Chicken Stands on One Leg

Continuing on, drop the right leg back to the rear, bend the knee and sit fully on it. The right arm also descends—as in Picture 72, Foot Diagram 81.

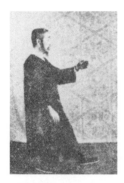

PICTURE 72

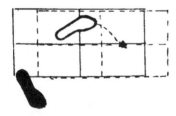

FOOT DIAGRAM 81

Simultaneously, raise the left elbow and left knee so the two connect, exactly as in the previous right-side posture. This is Left Golden Chicken Stands on One Leg—see Posture Twenty-Five, Foot Diagram 82.

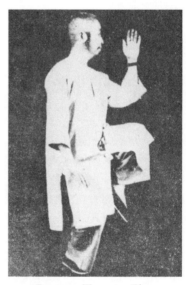

Posture Twenty-Five

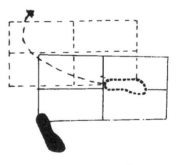

FOOT DIAGRAM 82

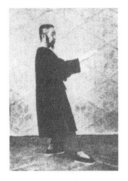

PICTURE 73

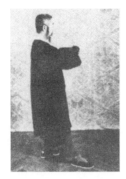

PICTURE 74

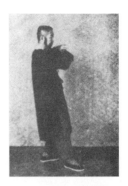

PICTURE 75

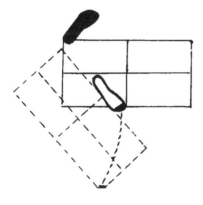

FOOT DIAGRAM 83

Twenty-Six: Separate Right and Left Leg

Drop your left leg back to the left-rear corner, bend the knee, and sit fully on it. Bring the right leg back, heel raised. Turn the left hand over and drop it as it follows the movement and descends. As you raise the right hand to meet the left hand, the two form a Left Roll-Back Posture—as in Picture 73, Foot Diagram 83.

The two arms roll back to the left-rear corner. The left arm momentates and circles from bottom to top; the right arm momentates down, eventually connecting with the left hand, under the left wrist. The two wrists intersect, both warding-off in front of the chest—as in Picture 74, the feet remain stationary.

Turn, the two arms rotate out—as in Picture 75. As you raise the right leg toward the right-front corner, the toes should be level with the instep as it slices forward. The knee and thigh should also be level. The two arms separate right and left, respectively, descending until they reach shoulder level. The right arm and right leg form a straight line. Note: In Posture Twenty-Six, my left arm is blocked from view. Please refer to the Left position of this posture for its proper placement. This is Separate Right Leg—see Posture Twenty-Six, Foot Diagram 84.

Continuing on, bring back the right foot while keeping the leg suspended. Then drop the right foot to the right-front cor-

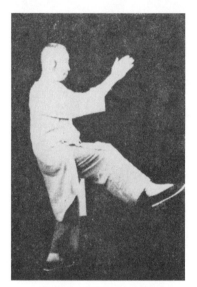

ner, bend the knee, and sit fully on it. The right arm simultaneously follows the waist/hip joint and moves back, turning over, under the left elbow. Next, roll back to the right side—as in Picture 76, Foot Diagram 85.

Posture Twenty-Six

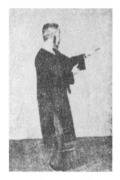

PICTURE 76

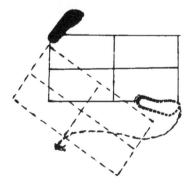

FOOT DIAGRAM 84

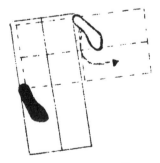

FOOT DIAGRAM 85

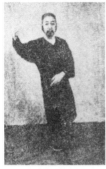
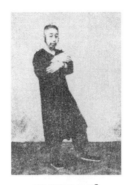
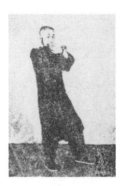

PICTURE 77   PICTURE 78   PICTURE 79

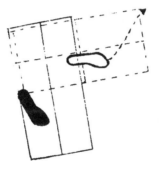

FOOT DIAGRAM 86

The right arm circles from bottom to top until it is level with the right shoulder and ear, while the left hand drops to the side of the right hip joint—as in Picture 77, the feet remain stationary.

The left arm descends while the right arm rises, and they meet in front with the two wrists connected. Meanwhile, the left foot takes one half-step to the left-front side—as in Picture 78, Foot Diagram 86.

Rotate the two wrists out—as in Picture 79, the feet remain stationary.

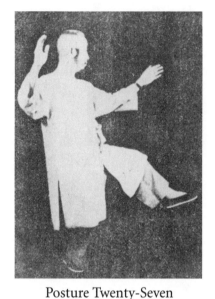

Raise the left leg following the waist/hip joint. The remaining moves are exactly the same as the previous posture. This is Separate Left Leg—see Posture Twenty-Seven, Foot Diagram 87.

Posture Twenty-Seven

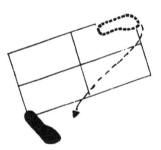

FOOT DIAGRAM 87

Twenty-Eight: Turn the Body, Kick

Proceeding from the previous posture, draw both arms and the left leg back in toward you. The left arm performs a Ward-Off

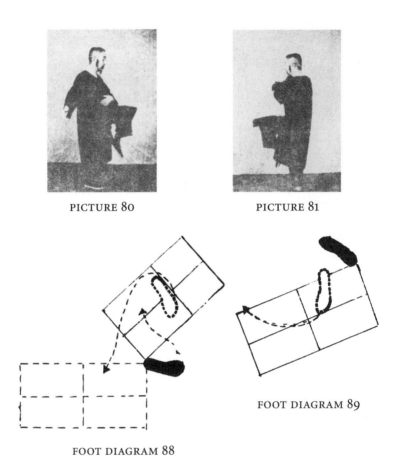

PICTURE 80

PICTURE 81

FOOT DIAGRAM 89

FOOT DIAGRAM 88

in front of your chest, while the right hand drops—as in Picture 80, Foot Diagram 88.

Raise the tip of the right foot and, following the waist/hip joint, turn toward the left rear 165 degrees. The left foot now faces the front left side. Turn the two arms out as in the previous posture, while the left leg hangs in mid-air—as in Picture 81, Foot Diagram 89.

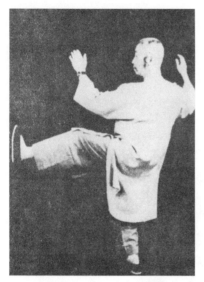

Posture Twenty-Eight

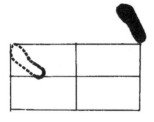

FOOT DIAGRAM 90

Continuing on, raise the left knee in toward the left elbow. The tip of the left foot rises and kicks forward with your heel. Open the two arms until the hands are level with the ears, in line with the left leg—see Posture Twenty-Eight, Foot Diagram 90. Note: Be careful to keep the heel steady when you pivot 360 degrees. The entire turn is based on the momentating positioning and turning of the right arm, which guides you much like a rudder. Only the right heel touches the ground as you turn.

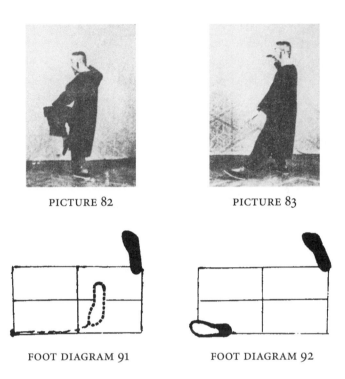

PICTURE 82   PICTURE 83

FOOT DIAGRAM 91   FOOT DIAGRAM 92

Brush Knee Twist Step, Left and Right

Continuing on, bring back the left arm and leg following the waist/hip joint, then place the left hand near the left knee. Drop the right hand next to the right ear—as in Picture 82, Foot Diagram 91.

Take a step forward with the left leg, heel first. The left hand brushes past the left knee, the right hand follows the waist/hip joint and slices forward—as in Picture 83, Foot Diagram 92.

Shift slowly onto the left leg, bend the knee, and sit on it. The left hand continues to brush until it is beside the left hip joint. The right hand follows the waist until the turn is com-

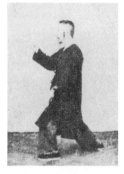

PICTURE 84

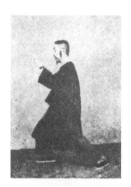

PICTURE 85

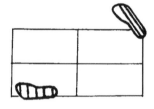

FOOT DIAGRAM 93

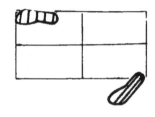

FOOT DIAGRAM 95

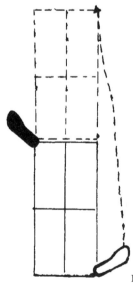

FOOT DIAGRAM 94

pleted, then sit on the wrist and erect the open hand. This is Brush Knee, Left—see Picture 84, Foot Diagram 93, 94.

Brush Knee Twist Step, Right, is the same as the previous posture—see Picture 85, Foot Diagram 95.

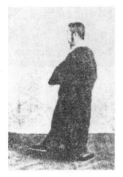

PICTURE 86

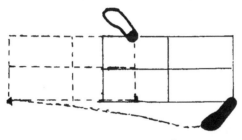

FOOT DIAGRAM 96

Twenty-Nine: Step Forward, Plant Fist

Proceeding from the previous posture, shift onto the left leg, bend the knee, and sit fully on it. Pivot the right foot out forty-five degrees. Drop the left wrist next to the right side of the short ribs. The right hand follows the position and momentates in a small circle, changes to a fist, and drops next to the right hip joint, Tiger Mouth pointing left. When the feet change from full to empty, the Tiger Mouth turns up—see Picture 86, Foot Diagram 96.

Shift onto the right leg, bend the knee, and sit fully on it. The left leg follows the momentum of the waist/hip joint, and takes one large step forward, heel first, then shifts slowly onto

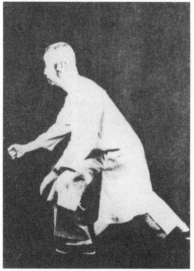

it. The right fist punches forward and down, as if you are planting your fist into the ground. Simultaneously, the left hand brushes the left knee—see Posture Twenty-Nine, Foot Diagram 97.

Posture Twenty-Nine

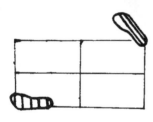

FOOT DIAGRAM 97

Step Forward, Grasp the Sparrow's Tail, Single Whip

Proceeding on, Ward-Off, Roll-Back, Press, Push, and Single Whip have all been explained before. I will include illustrations of these postures. See Pictures 87 through 100, and Foot Diagrams 98 through 109.

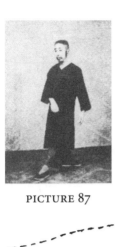

PICTURE 87

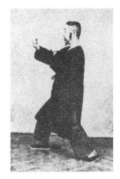

PICTURE 88

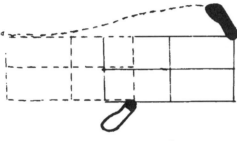

FOOT DIAGRAM 98

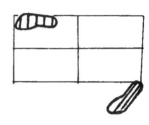

FOOT DIAGRAM 99

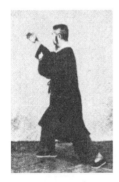

PICTURE 89

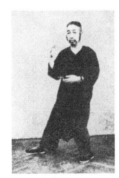

PICTURE 90

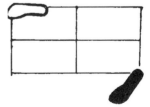

FOOT DIAGRAM 100

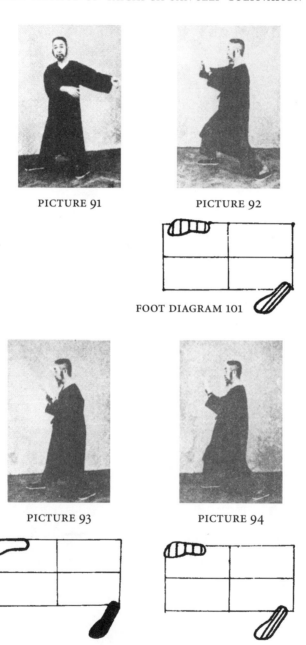

PICTURE 91

PICTURE 92

FOOT DIAGRAM 101

PICTURE 93

PICTURE 94

FOOT DIAGRAM 102

FOOT DIAGRAM 103

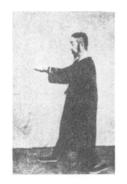

PICTURE 95

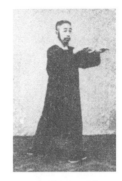

PICTURE 96

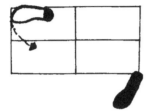

FOOT DIAGRAM 104

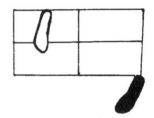

FOOT DIAGRAM 105

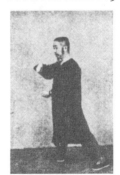

PICTURE 97

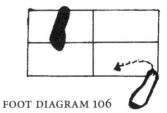

FOOT DIAGRAM 106

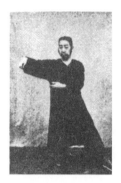

PICTURE 98

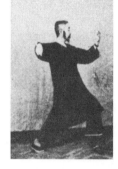

PICTURE 99

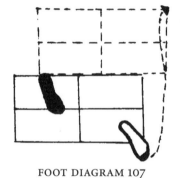

FOOT DIAGRAM 107

FOOT DIAGRAM 108

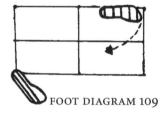

PICTURE 100

FOOT DIAGRAM 109

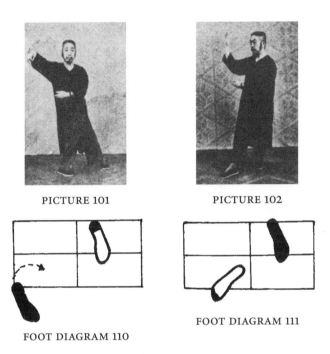

PICTURE 101

PICTURE 102

FOOT DIAGRAM 111

FOOT DIAGRAM 110

Thirty through Thirty-Three:
Fair Lady Works the Shuttle

Proceeding on from the last posture, shift onto the right leg, bend the knee, and sit fully on it. Raise the left foot tip and pivot inward. The left hand turns over following the waist/hip joint, momentating under the right armpit—as in Picture 101, Foot Diagram 110.

Shift onto the left leg, bend the knee, and sit fully on it. Raise the right heel and follow the waist/hip joint as they turn to the right-rear corner. Simultaneously, relax open the right hanging hand and place it erect, palm in. The left hand assists under the right elbow—as in Picture 102, Foot Diagram 111.

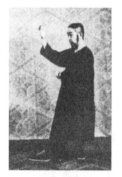

PICTURE 103

Continuing on, raise the right leg and turn the tip of the foot about fifteen degrees to the right-front corner—as in Picture 103, Foot Diagram 112.

Next, shift onto the right leg, bend the knee, and sit fully on it. Take a large step with the left foot to the left-front corner, bend the knee, and sit on it. Simultaneously, raise the left arm following the waist/hip joint, palm out, protecting the left side of the forehead. Drop the right hand as it pushes forward, following the inner left forearm, palm out. This is Fair Lady Works the Shuttle, One—see Posture Thirty, Foot Diagram 113.

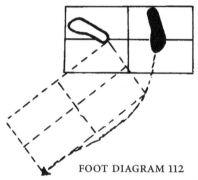

FOOT DIAGRAM 112

Continuing on, shift onto the right leg, bend the knee, and sit fully on it. Raise the left toes and pivot 130 degrees to the right rear following the waist. Shift onto the left leg, bend the

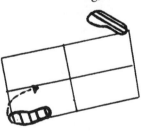

FOOT DIAGRAM 113

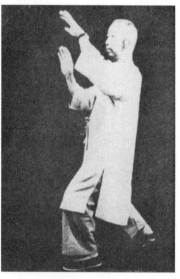

Posture Thirty

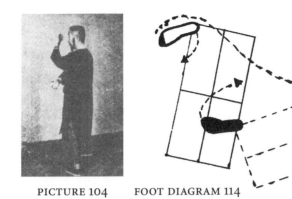

PICTURE 104   FOOT DIAGRAM 114

knee, and sit fully on it. The erect open left hand turns palm in, opposite your face, the right hand turns palm up—as in Picture 104, Foot Diagram 114.

Continuing on, raise the right heel and, following the turn and momentum of the waist, take a large step to the right rear corner, about 270 degrees, heel first. Gradually bend the knee and sit fully on the leg. Raise the right arm to protect the right side of the forehead, palm out. The left erect hand follows the right hand and descends, pushing forward near the right elbow. The hand turns out as it pushes forward, while the left foot pivots in. This is Fair Lady Works the Shuttle, Two—see Posture Thirty-One, Foot Diagram 115.

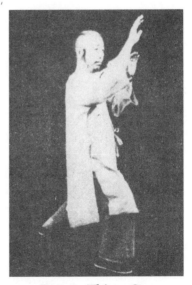

Posture Thirty-One

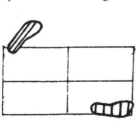

FOOT DIAGRAM 115

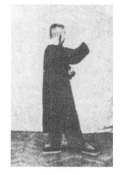

Continuing on, shift onto the left leg, bend the knee, and sit fully on it. Bring the right foot back a little to the left side, and point the toes to the right. At the same time, turn the right hand over, palm in. The left hand also turns over and assists under the right elbow—as in Picture 105, Foot Diagram 116.

Continuing on, the left foot takes a large step to the left-front corner, heel first. Slowly bend the knee and sit fully on it. The right foot turns with the waist to the left front, coming together with the left hip joint. The remaining shuttle movements of the elbows are exactly the same as the previous Posture One. This is Fair Lady Works the

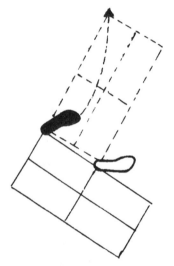

FOOT DIAGRAM 116

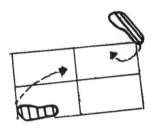

FOOT DIAGRAM 117

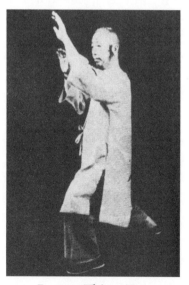

Posture Thirty-Two

104

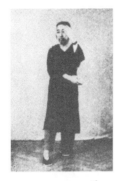

PICTURE 106

Shuttle, Three—see Posture Thirty-Two, Foot Diagram 117.

Next, shift onto the right leg, bend the knee, and sit fully on it. Raise the left toes and, following the waist/hip joint, turn as far as you can to the right, then sit fully on the leg. Shift onto the left leg, raise the right heel, and momentate it back with the waist/hip joint. Simultaneously, the left hand moves to the inner left side and the palm turns under the left elbow—as in Picture 106, Foot Diagram 118.

The remaining positions are the same as Posture Two. This is Fair Lady Works the Shuttle, Four—see Posture Thirty-Three, Foot Diagram 119.

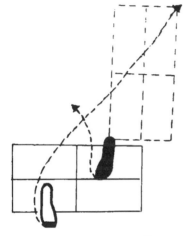

FOOT DIAGRAM 118

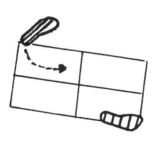

FOOT DIAGRAM 119

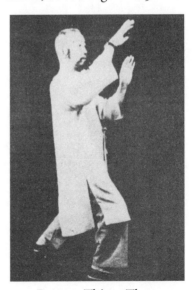

Posture Thirty-Three

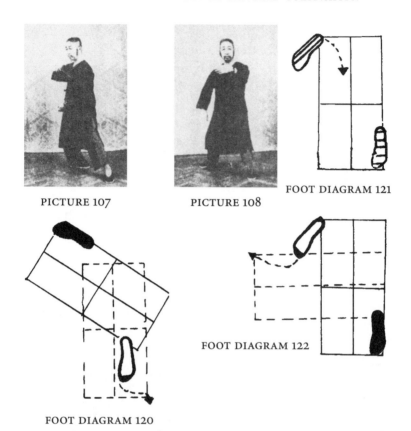

PICTURE 107   PICTURE 108

FOOT DIAGRAM 121

FOOT DIAGRAM 122

FOOT DIAGRAM 120

Grasping the Sparrow's Tail to Single Squatting Whip

Proceeding on, turn the waist/hip joint to the left front, raise the right heel, and momentate it back. Simultaneously, as you drop the two elbows, the left open hand assists under the right elbow. Together they appear to be holding something—as in Picture 107, Foot Diagram 120.

Next, place the left foot one half-step to the left front. Bend the knee and sit on it. The left arm performs a Ward-Off, and the right hand drops to the side of the right hip joint. This is Left Ward-Off—see Picture 108, Foot Diagram 121.

The following postures, Right Ward-Off, Roll-Back, Press, Push, and Single Squatting-Whip have all been explained above. Refer to Pictures 109 through 134 and Foot Diagrams 122 through 138.

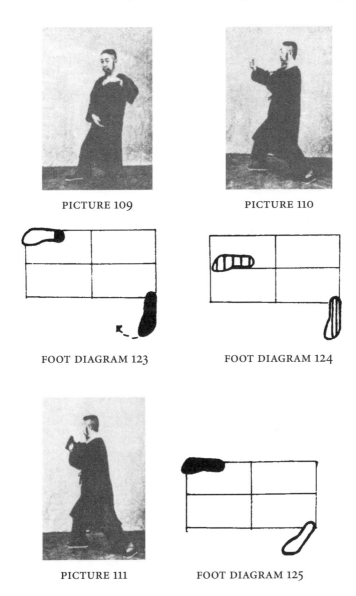

PICTURE 109 PICTURE 110

FOOT DIAGRAM 123 FOOT DIAGRAM 124

PICTURE 111 FOOT DIAGRAM 125

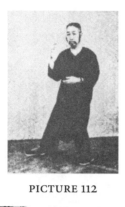

PICTURE 112

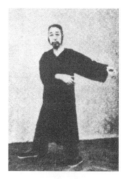

PICTURE 113

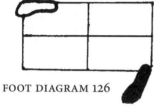

FOOT DIAGRAM 126

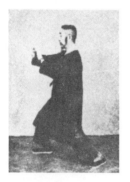

PICTURE 114

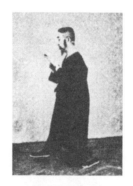

PICTURE 115

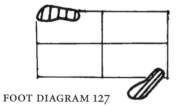

FOOT DIAGRAM 127

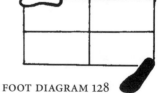

FOOT DIAGRAM 128

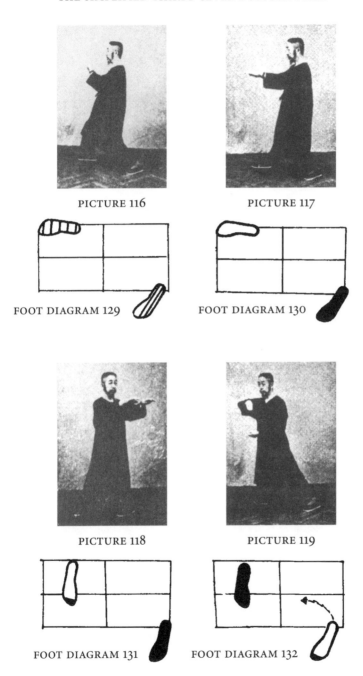

PICTURE 116

PICTURE 117

FOOT DIAGRAM 129

FOOT DIAGRAM 130

PICTURE 118

PICTURE 119

FOOT DIAGRAM 131

FOOT DIAGRAM 132

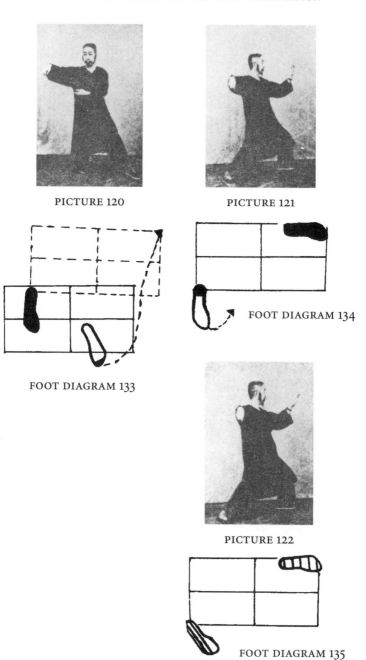

PICTURE 120

PICTURE 121

FOOT DIAGRAM 134

FOOT DIAGRAM 133

PICTURE 122

FOOT DIAGRAM 135

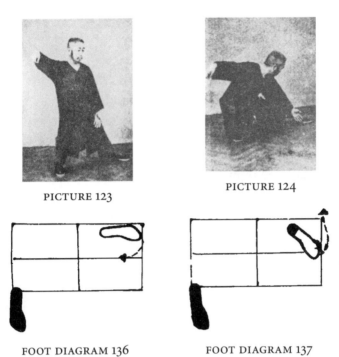

PICTURE 123

PICTURE 124

FOOT DIAGRAM 136

FOOT DIAGRAM 137

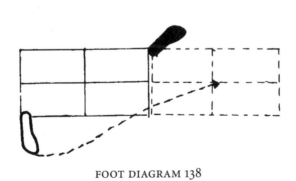

FOOT DIAGRAM 138

Thirty-Four: The Seven Stars Step Forward

Proceeding on, pivot the left foot tip ninety degrees left. Shift onto the left leg, bend the knee, and sit fully on it. Simultaneously, the right foot takes one full step forward, toes touching the ground. Raise the left hand to form a fist in front of the chest. Raise the right hanging hand and form a fist, intersecting under the left wrist. This is Seven Stars Step Forward—see Posture Thirty-Four, Foot Diagram 139.

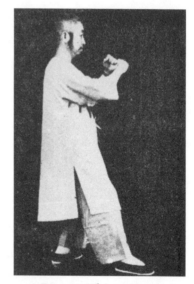

Posture Thirty-Four

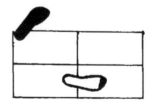

FOOT DIAGRAM 139

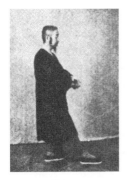

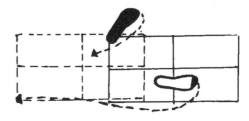

FOOT DIAGRAM 140

PICTURE 125

Thirty-Five: Step Back, Ride the Tiger

Continuing on, relax open the two wrists. The left open hand turns down, the right turns up, keeping the two wrists connected—as in Picture 125, Foot Diagram 140. The right leg steps back one large step, then bend the knee and sit fully on it. Bring the left foot back a little, toes touching. The two forearms open, and the right arm circles up and stands erect outside the right shoulder, palm forward. The left hand descends and brushes the knee, protecting the left side of the crotch— see Posture Thirty-Five, Foot Diagram 141.

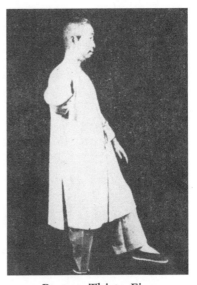

Posture Thirty-Five

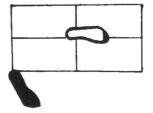

FOOT DIAGRAM 141

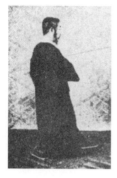

PICTURE 126

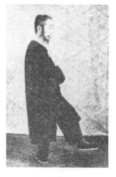

PICTURE 127

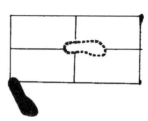

FOOT DIAGRAM 142

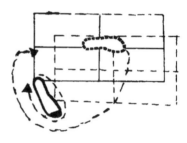

FOOT DIAGRAM 143

Thirty-Six: Turn the Body, Sweep the Lotus

Continuing on, turn the waist/hip joint left. Drop the right arm and momentate it to the left, resting it between the left short-ribs and left hip joint. The left hand follows and turns a little to the left, palm forward—as in Picture 126, the feet remain stationary.

Next, raise the left foot and let it hang in midair—as in Picture 127, Foot Diagram 142 and 143.

The left arm and left leg ride the posture as you turn to the right circling with momentum 360 degrees on your right toes, just like a toy top. The right heel must remain stable—that is extremely important! The left foot drops at a forty-five-degree

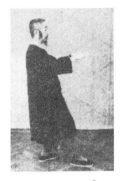

angle from the front, the tip slightly raised. The two arms momentate to the front chest area, palms down. This is called Turn the Body—see Picture 128, Foot Diagram 144.

Next, relax the left waist/hip joint, and sit fully on the left leg. Raise the right leg following this position and circle it from right to left in front of the crotch. The toes should brush the tips

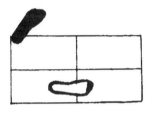

FOOT DIAGRAM 144

of your fingers. This is called Sweep the Lotus—see Posture Thirty-Six, Foot Diagram 145.

Note: There are several points to remember with this posture. First, keep the two arms steady. Second, do not force the leg to sweep the fingers. If you cannot reach them, let it be. This ability comes naturally with practice.

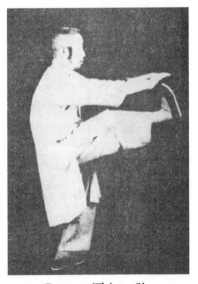

Posture Thirty-Six

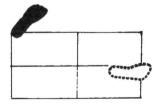

FOOT DIAGRAM 145

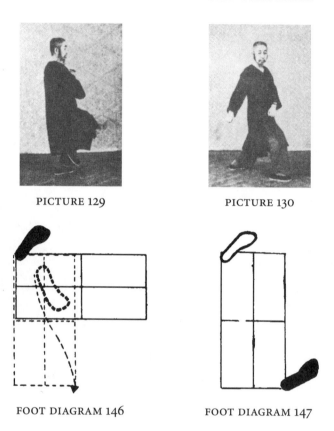

PICTURE 129

PICTURE 130

FOOT DIAGRAM 146

FOOT DIAGRAM 147

Thirty-Seven: Bend the Bow, Shoot the Tiger

After you sweep your fingers, draw the right leg back next to the left calf. Pull the two arms next to the left short-ribs area. The left hand turns wrist down, the right wrist turns sideways and assists near the left waist—as in Picture 129, Foot Diagram 146.

Next, drop the right leg to the right-front corner, bend the knee, and sit fully on it. Drop the two hands and form fists, momentating to the right-rear corner—as in Picture 130, Foot Diagram 147.

Next, the two arms follow the position and circle from bottom to top. The right fist turns up to the right ear, Tiger's Mouth pointing left. The left fist drops to the side of the right short-ribs area, the left Tiger's Mouth aligned with the Right Tiger's Mouth. This is called Bend the Bow, Shoot the Tiger—see Posture Thirty-Seven, Foot Diagram 148.

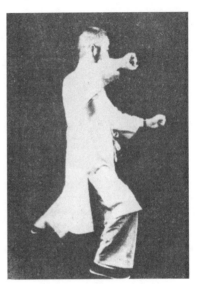

Posture Thirty-Seven

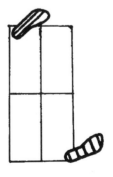

FOOT DIAGRAM 148

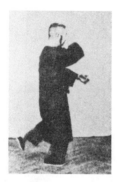

PICTURE 131

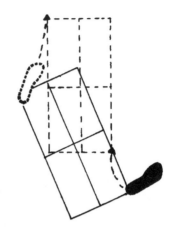

FOOT DIAGRAM 149

Step Forward, Block, Parry, Punch, Cross Hands, and Return to Origin

Proceeding on, lift the left foot about one inch. The left hand relaxes open and moves to protect under the right elbow, preparing for a Roll-Back—as in Picture 131, Foot Diagram 149.

Drop the left foot, bend the knee, and sit fully on it. The left hand descends into a Roll-Back. The proceeding moves, Step Forward, Block, Parry, Punch, Cross Hands, and Return to Origin, have all been explained before. See Pictures 132 through 143, and Foot Diagrams, 150 through 160. They are all arranged in proper sequence.

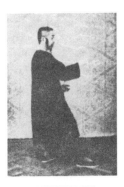

PICTURE 132

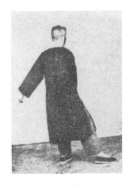

PICTURE 133

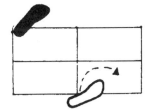

FOOT DIAGRAM 150

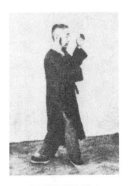

PICTURE 134

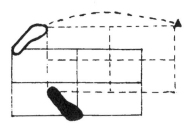

FOOT DIAGRAM 151

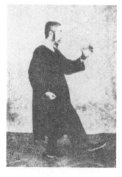

PICTURE 135

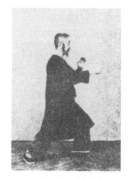

PICTURE 136

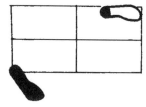

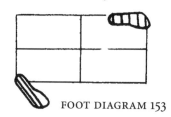

FOOT DIAGRAM 153

FOOT DIAGRAM 152

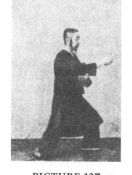

PICTURE 137

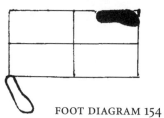

FOOT DIAGRAM 154

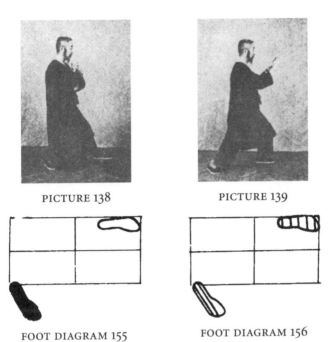

PICTURE 138

PICTURE 139

FOOT DIAGRAM 155

FOOT DIAGRAM 156

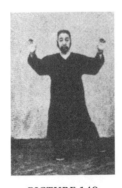

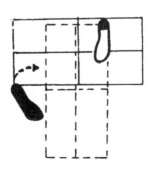

PICTURE 140

FOOT DIAGRAM 157

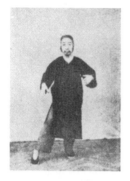

PICTURE 141

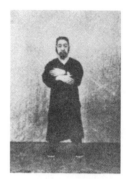

PICTURE 142

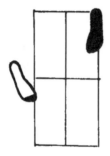

FOOT DIAGRAM 158

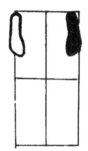

FOOT DIAGRAM 159

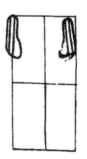

FOOT DIAGRAM 160

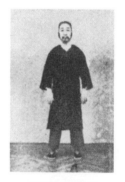

PICTURE 143

Afterword

SIXTY TO SEVENTY PERCENT of all beginning taichi enthusi-
asts hurriedly finish a superficial study of the form and
blithely proclaim their understanding. They procrastinate in
their daily practice and eventually stop altogether. In reality,
they enter a treasure trove and exit empty-handed. Though
taichi is a golden elixir of health, this elixir does not come in
pill form. The *I Ching* says, "As nature is constantly creatively
active, so too the noble man never rests in improving himself."
This means that self-improvement requires constant work. Only
then will you emulate nature's creativity. When this is possible,
your practice of taichi will bestow its benefits as an elixir for
health. This is why I place perseverance first and foremost among
the three faults to be eliminated first.

Thirty years ago I wrote in the Afterword to my *Thirteen
Treatises* that taichi was perfectly suited to females' nature and
that it was more important to them than for men. I also said
that taichi could transform your disposition, and that it sur-
passed every other exercise. Parents concerned about the future
health of their offspring should practice taichi around the home.
This will imperceptibly influence their children's view of the
art, and they will one day enjoy practicing it. Taichi is not merely
a wonderful prescription for health; it molds both character
and nature while self-cultivation is unconsciously accomplished.

I once composed a poem with a verse that read, "Where will I find the eloquence, to adequately praise taichi?" In this respect I emulate Vimalakirti's compassion for the sick and Confucius' spirit for universal commiseration.

Examples of Taichi Philosophy
in Classical Literature

The *I Ching*

The noble man is creatively active throughout the day, and beset with cares at night. No blame.

As nature is constantly creatively active, the noble man never rests improving himself.

Arrogance is knowing when to press forward but not draw back; understanding existence but not annihilation; thinking of gains but not loss.

Success comes through *shih-chung*, synchronicity. I do not seek the student, the student must seek me.

Give up resistance, accept following.

The Abysmal is double danger.

There is a proper time to decrease the hard and increase the soft. Increase, decrease, full, and empty; all must proceed according to the proper time.

The Confucian *I Ching*, *(Hsi Tzu Ch'uan)*

Heaven is superior, earth is inferior; Ch'ien and K'un are thus determined.

The firm and yielding interact with each other, the eight trigrams succeed one another.

By what is simple and easy, all the principles under heaven are understood.

Change and transformation are the images of progression and regression.

Affairs are what penetrate change; spirit is the unfathomable aspect of yin/yang.

Understanding the Tao of change, comprehends the actions of the divine!

The divine can hurry without haste and foretell the future.

The Receptive is like a closing gate, the Creative is its opening; change is the alternation of the two.

In the *I Ching* there is Taichi; this produces the Two Aspects, yin and yang; these produce the Four Primary Images; these produce the Eight Trigrams.

The firm and yielding push each other, change proceeds from within.

When something runs to its end, it changes. By changing it achieves continuity.

Lao Tzu's *Tao Teh Ching*

Empty the mind, fill the abdomen; gentle the will, strengthen the bones. (Chapter # 3)

Empty, yet inexhaustible; move, and more issues forth. (#5)

Ch'i lingers in wisps, use it without haste. (#6)

The sage puts himself last and ends up ahead, he keeps himself outside worldly affairs and thus maintains himself. (#7)

Concentrate your ch'i to become soft and young. (#10)

With no sense of self, what can injure you? (#13)

Small amounts are attainable, too much is confusing. So the sage embraces the One, and becomes a model for all the world. (#22)

If you wish to shrink something, you must first stretch it; to weaken something you must first strengthen it; if you want to eradicate something you must first erect it; if you want to take something you must first give: this is called understanding the subtle. (#36)

The Tao moves by returning, it functions through softness. (#40)

When a superior man hears the Tao, he practices it tirelessly; when a mediocre man hears of it, he occasionally practices it; when a lowly man hears of it, he laughs. If he did not laugh, it would not be the Tao. (#41)

The hard die an unnatural death. (#42)

The softest thing in the world overcomes the hardest thing in the world. (#43)

Those who excel in living can travel without meeting a tiger or rhino; in battle no weapon penetrates their armor. The rhino has no place to gore, the tiger feels nowhere to claw, the soldier finds nowhere to stab. Why is this? Because they have no fear of death. (#50)

Motherly love brings courage. (#67)

Good men are not aggressive, good soldiers do not become angry. (#68)

The stiff and hard are followers of death, the soft and supple are disciples of life. (#76)

Water is the softest thing in the world, yet when attacking the hard and strong, nothing overcomes it. (#78)

The Yellow Emperor's Classic on Internal Medicine

The Yellow Emperor asked the Supreme Teacher, "I have heard that the ancients lived over one hundred years and yet remained active. Nowadays, men half that age are invalids. Is the world changing? Or has man lost the teachings?"

Ch'i Po answered, "The ancients understood the Tao. They patterned themselves after the yin/yang, and lived in harmony through divination. Their eating habits were temperate, their lifestyle regulated, and they never overworked themselves needlessly. They thus maintained body and spirit, living out their ordained life span. At one hundred they died."

The Yellow Emperor said, "From early times, understanding nature was the foundation of existence. Based upon the yin/yang, placed within heaven and earth and the six directions, its ch'i fills the Nine Provinces, the Nine Body Orifices, the Five Viscera, and the Twelve Joints; all are permeated with nature's ch'i.

"Yin and yang is the Tao of heaven and earth. They are the principles of all living things, the parents of change. They are the root and beginning of life and death, and the depot of divine clarity."

"The ancient sages transmitted the teachings of essence *(ching)* and spirit *(shen)*, of swallowing nature's ch'i, and penetrating divine clarity."

"Those who follow the way escape old age intact."

"In repose of perfect emptiness, the True Ch'i will follow. With essence and spirit guarded within, how can illnesses be caught? Quiet the will and decrease desires, then the mind will be comfortable and unafraid, and you can work without being tired."

"The sage set forth the yin/yang, so their sinews harmonized with the vessels, marrow hardened their bones, and blood flowed smoothly with ch'i."